MIND/BODY TECHNIQUES FOR ASPERGER'S SYNDROME

of related interest

The Complete Guide to Asperger's Syndrome
Tony Attwood
ISBN 978 1 84310 495 7

Yoga for Children with Autism Spectrum Disorders
A Step-by-Step Guide for Parents and Caregivers
Dion E. Betts and Stacey W. Betts
Forewords by Louise Goldberg, Registered Yoga Teacher and Joshua S. Betts
ISBN 978 1 84310 817 7

Integrated Yoga
Yoga with a Sensory Integrative Approach
Nicole Cuomo
ISBN 978 1 84310 862 7

Creative Expressive Activities and Asperger's Syndrome
Social and Emotional Skills and Positive Life Goals for Adolescents and Young Adults
Judith Martinovich
ISBN 978 1 84310 812 2

MIND/BODY TECHNIQUES FOR ASPERGER'S SYNDROME

THE WAY OF THE PATHFINDER

RON RUBIO

FOREWORDS BY
IRENE BRODY AND ANTHONY CASTROGIOVANNI

Jessica Kingsley Publishers
London and Philadelphia

First published in 2008
by Jessica Kingsley Publishers
116 Pentonville Road
London N1 9JB, UK
and
400 Market Street, Suite 400
Philadelphia, PA 19106, USA

www.jkp.com

Library of Congress Cataloging in Publication Data
Rubio, Ron, 1957-
Mind/body techniques for Asperger's syndrome : way of the pathfinder / Ron Rubio ; foreword by Irene Brody.
 p. ; cm.
Includes bibliographical references.
 ISBN-13: 978-1-84310-875-7 (pbk. : alk. paper) 1. Asperger's syndrome--Exercise therapy. 2. Asperger's syndrome--Patients--Rehabilitation. 3. Martial arts--Therapeutic use. 4. Holistic medicine. 5. Mind and body. I. Title.
 [DNLM: 1. Asperger Syndrome--therapy. 2. Exercise Therapy--methods. 3. Holistic Health. 4. Martial Arts--psychology. WM 203.5 R896m 2008]
 RC553.A88R83 2008
 616.85'8832062--dc22

2007031527

British Library Cataloguing in Publication Data
A CIP catalogue record for this book is available from the British Library

ISBN 978 1 84310 875 7

Printed and bound in the United States by
Thomson-Shore Inc. (tbc)

This book is dedicated to my maternal grandfather,
who was a true warrior, a man of his word
and a person of a world and age gone by.

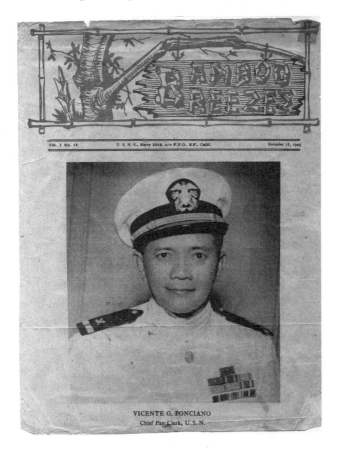

Vincente G. Ponciano—first Filipino officer
in the United States Navy
Veteran of World War 2—
Pacific Theater of Operations
Bataan Death March Survivor

Contents

Preface *9*

Acknowledgments *12*

Foreword by Irene Brody, Ph.D 14

Foreword by Anthony Castrogiovanni, Ph.D 17

1. Introduction to Core Concepts of Pathfinder
    Mentoring 21
2. The Breath Foundation: Being Grounded 39
3. Mindfulness: Taming "the Chattering Mind" 55
4. Standing on Your Own Two Feet 64
5. Posture, Presence, and Extension 87
6. The Power of Movement 112
7. The Rites of Passage 143

Bibliography *147*

Index *150*

Preface

Relationship—sacredness—warriorship—mentorship

This manual, *Mind/Body Techniques for Asperger's Syndrome: The Way of the Pathfinder*, on one level is about the Pathfinder holistic mind/body model that supports the evolving person aged eight years and up, who is challenged with any or all of the following: autism, learning disabilities, Obsessive Compulsive Disorder (OCD), Attention Deficit Hyperactivity Disorder (ADHD), Post Traumatic Stress Disorder (PTSD) or Asperger's Syndrome (AS). On another level, this manual is about building bridges of communication between two people that stimulate creative thinking for developing a meaningful and positive relationship. Most importantly, this manual speaks about honoring the profound sacredness of each moment—of each second of life—that is expressed through the paradigm of a holistic warriorship.

In human relationships there is the initial "point of contact" that will evolve in the direction of either a deeper, more meaningful connection of true listening and sharing interaction, or that will spiral down the superficial and pretentious path of "filler and fluff" communication until the conversation fades and diminishes like the lingering light of a blown-out candle. Within the initial moments of point of contact, building an interface—a bridge of honesty and trust, strength with sensitivity, humility and empathy, honor, and respect—is crucial for success.

In the martial arts, this point of contact is the moment of blending, guiding, staying "sticky" with, controlling, dominating, destroying, or finding a harmonious resolution. As in any relationship, the initial martial art encounter is open to the many various responses that are dictated by the intention and intensity of the energy or action directed at the martial artist. I have found in my own studies in the martial arts that the point of contact is the opportunity for me to choose to blend, stay sticky with, and find harmonious resolution with my practice partner. When working with a client with AS, for instance, I use the same strategy—blend, stay sticky with, and find harmonious resolution.

The initial moments of point of contact with a room of 40 dance students or the private client is the same: establish trust, honor, and respect by showing that it is a two-way street in which trust, honor, and respect are offered and received by me and any student. For all the information and wisdom that can be offered by a teacher to be successfully implemented and used by a student hinges on a solid relationship. I hold the moment of creating the interface between me and another person to be a sacred moment that can never be taken back once passed.

Here the word "sacred" is used to describe the precious and revered holiness that is present in all beings. Sacredness is present and alive in every expression and texture of life. To see the very fine as well as the large details that surround you; to smell the subtle fragrances of the vibrant life in the cool evenings; to feel the scorch of the sun, the sharpness of bitter cold, the flaying of an intense wind—every nuance that the physical world offers you in every moment and every second of your life. The honoring of sacredness is deeply intertwined in the fibers that make up the foundation of the holistic warriorship paradigm that I mentor and live by.

The study of this holistic warriorship is one of contemplating one's inner faith of what is sacred—what is holy, the virtue of having compassion for others—which in turn is expressing compassion for oneself, the capacity of one's strength under fire, a fearlessness in the face of changing situations, and the willingness to forgive and heal.

Warriors honor sacredness for they are aware of how precious life is and that pure service must be free of fear and doubt in order to be effective and to survive whatever one faces. Japanese warriors, the *samurai*, faced their deaths daily with complete acceptance in order to live their lives of service without fear. The indigenous warriors of the North America plains had a saying, "It is a good day to die," as they prepared for battle. To me this said, "Live life without fear."

When the Persian King Xerses in 480 BC observed from a distance the Spartan warriors jovially bathing in the waters before him, combing and braiding their long hair, and grooming themselves before a decisive three-day battle for the Gates of Thermopylae, he was confused. Why were these outnumbered elite Greek warriors not quaking before the might of his vast army and fleeing for safety? Why were they grooming themselves so meticulously as if it was just another day on the military parade grounds? Xerxes had in his employment an exiled Spartan king who provided an answer, "O Mighty King Xerxes," he said, "they are preparing for their deaths!" In the ensuing battle the Spartans and their Greek allies died to the man defending not just "property," but the idea of pure service and dedication to a mission that was placed upon them. This ancient warrior story had a profound effect on me as a young boy. The thought of such fearlessness, boldness, and audacity displayed in the face of such overwhelming odds inspired a resonating way of thinking in me.

Which brings me to speak of mentoring. Mentoring is a path of service. A mentor is entrusted by a child's parents to teach their evolving child the responsibilities of adulthood and to help create and develop the child's personal path that best expresses their strengths for a fulfilled life in the community, the tribe, and the family to which they belong. A mentor says what needs to be said without all the emotional charges of resistance. To mentor a "high maintenance" and challenging young person to a place of personal inner safety, self-confidence, and faith in oneself, the Pathfinder mentor must face the mentee's deepest demons, fears, trauma, and rage with fearlessness, compassion, boldness, and creativity.

A Pathfinder mentor creates paths and options where none may exist. Historically, military pathfinders were specially trained warriors who infiltrated deep into enemy territory, way ahead of the main force, to find, create, and secure a logistical point of entry amid the enemy position for their comrades-in-arms to follow.

This manual is an introduction to the Pathfinder training. It speaks about sacredness and holiness, honor and respect, presence, empowerment, communication, building relationships, leadership, courage and boldness, compassion and empathy, tolerance and patience.

It is a gift of service.

Ron Rubio
Catskills Mountains of New York

Acknowledgments

I would like to give thanks to Great Spirit Great Universe for all the gifts bestowed upon me through the love of my family, my friends, and my community. I thank you.

I bow graciously to the Alvin Ailey Dance Company and school for all the inspiration, vision, grace, power, elegance, and self-awareness that I was taught as a full-time scholarship student there (1979–1981).

Madame Zena Rommett, I thank you so much for offering a work scholarship to a crazy young dancer. Your innovative techniques of body alignment using ballet floor barre exercises made a strong and enlightened dancer out of me.

All the lovingly demanding New York city dance teachers, choreographers, and fellow dancers who had to put up with me all those years, I thank you.

Through the years, I have been honored to be a student of the martial arts under the tutelage of some very extraordinary and generous human beings.

I give great respect and gratitude to my *aikido* teacher—Sensei Yoshimitsu Yamada 8th dan—Chief Instructor of the New York Aikikai and Chairman of the United States Aikido Federation.

I deeply acknowledge the teaching of my *aikido* mentors through the years—Sempai Stuart Robert Allen, senior teachers of The New York Aikikai: Harvey Konigsberg 7th dan (Woodstock Aikido), Hal Lerman 7th dan (Aikido of Park Slope), Jane Oseki 7th dan, Steve Pimpsler 7th dan, the late Mitsunari Kanai Sensei of the New England Aikikai and the late

Mike Mamura Sensei of Milwaukee Aikido. I would like to offer gratitude to Mitsugi Saotome Sensei 8th dan, Chairman of the Aikido School of Ueshiba, and the senior teachers of the Aikido Shobukan Dojo of Washington, DC.

I give thanks and gratitude to my martial art teachers—*capoeria* master, Bira Almeida Mestre Acordeon; self-defense close combat expert, John Perkins; and ex-Heavyweight Boxing Champion of the World, the late Floyd Patterson, for all the free boxing lessons and a warm loving heart.

Thank you to Mr Burrill Crohn for his DVD filming and editing work.

Thank you very much, Jessica Stevens, Commissioning Editor of Jessica Kingsley Publishers, for your help and support.

Thank you, Jessica Kingsley Publishers, for the opportunity to present my work and be of service to others.

Foreword

One of the biggest needs of the autism spectrum community is finding therapists with related experience and knowledge. When I attend Autism Spectrum Disorder (ASD) conferences, what I hear directly from the mouths of those with autism and Asperger's Syndrome (AS) is, "Please help us find therapists who understand who we are, what we need, and how to communicate this information and learning to us."

Ron Rubio is one of those people. He has developed a unique and innovative therapy that addresses the needs of the ASD community, and he delivers it in a way that is effective, inspirational, and transformative. His clients walk away in a whole new manner, and I mean that literally, for they truly walk differently! Not only do they stand and move in new ways, they also talk, relate, and behave differently in the world. They find confidence in themselves they never experienced before. They find courage they never knew they had. And they never forget what they have learned, because it becomes an ingrained part of their bodies, minds, and spirits. Clients return to him after several years reporting that they continue to use what he has taught them. He is a true mentor on every level, and the proof is in the brave young men who have been mentored by him over the years. The changes that occur have been noted by teachers, parents, and most especially, by the clients themselves.

One of the most important questions before us today is what forms of therapy are truly helpful and effective? After many years in the field, leading social skills groups, counseling individuals, consulting with schools, and educating parents, here are my answers. As with any successful therapy, the relationship between the therapist and the client is paramount. Building that relationship with ASD people takes a different route from either the traditional "sit-down-and-talk" therapy, or the "play-with-sand-and-toys-and-I'll-watch-and-interpret" therapy. Therapy for the ASD community must be direct, concrete, non-verbal as well as verbal, and personal. You need to give more of yourself, show more of yourself, and be more engaging, hopefully even funny. In other words, you must be a mentor, and in the broadest way possible. You are a model of what it means to be a human being in connection with others in the world we live in. You must model and teach all aspects of this, from the basics of self-regulation, coping with stress, using flexibility in thinking, social skills, hygiene, daily living skills, right up to developing character.

In order to engage, a therapist or mentor working with ASD people must be able to use their interests to motivate them, as motivation itself is often a therapeutic challenge. One of the reasons Mr. Rubio's approach is effective is because he uses the paradigm of the warrior archetype. Besides the fact that the warrior is a concept that can teach many character traits, the warrior is also an ideal that many young people with autism and Asperger's can relate to, identify with, and be motivated by. How many young men and women with Asperger's can be found playing electronic games with fierce warriors and gruesome foes, or show an interest in military history and weaponry? Or perhaps I should ask, how many cannot be found thus engaged? And even for those whose interests lie elsewhere, the warrior concept is often one that is easily grasped as a metaphor for any young person struggling through life with the odds against them.

In order to be effective, the therapist must remediate the low self-esteem that is so common to the ASD community as a result of years of bullying and social exclusion, poor motor coordination, challenging organizational skills, and chronic anxiety. The therapeutic method cannot simply be one of reassuring or highlighting strengths, as in the too much used "But you're so smart." This ends up being a compensatory mechanism that falls apart under duress. Rather, a mentor teaches new skills, sets up new challenges, and instigates the mentees to tackle them until successful. Self-esteem comes from real accomplishments, from knowing one can overcome, and from having these achievements reflected in the eyes and words of those around one.

Finally, and by no means least, therapy with the ASD community has to incorporate a holistic integration that includes the body, mind, breath, and spirit/will/soul. As the first noted observer of Asperger's Syndrome, Hans Asperger himself pointed out the clumsy, uncoordinated physicality of this portion of the ASD community. And even though many autistic people have good physical coordination, they do not always link this ability to the rest of their being, such as being able to ground themselves through their body and breath when they are stressed, or to the way they present themselves to others socially. It is one thing to teach someone how to throw a ball in a gym class, how to start a conversation in a speech class, and how to think about a problem in a philosophy class. For a neuro-typical person, this style of learning might be ok because they can put all the pieces together on their own if need be. For those with ASD, the world is often experienced as being broken up into so many little bits and pieces. Getting started, putting it all together, in a workable sequence, in many situations with many variables, now there's the sticking point!

This book offers a technique that connects these dots. For example, breathing exercises are taught not just to release stress, they are taught to create a sense of wholeness, a new relationship to oneself and to others. In each and every exercise in this book, the mentee is entreated to activate every aspect of their being. At first glance, the exercises appear simple. And, indeed, in some ways they are; however, as one delves deeper into the work, one discovers that there is a lot more than meets the eye. In fact, I would be surprised if anyone reading this book, whether on the autistic spectrum or not, is not affected in some way themselves. If you truly want to understand how effective this method is, try the exercises yourself. Read, breathe, do, and enjoy!

Irene Brody, Ph.D.
Psychologist in private practice specializing in children,
adolescents, and adults with Asperger's Syndrome, Shokan, NY

Foreword

When I was a child, the genetic roll of the dice was very kind to me. I was a physically robust child—larger and more muscular at all stages than the developmental charts reported as average and, luckily for me, my size was accompanied by an equal helping of coordination. This led, with little effort on my part, to standing out in all manner of physical activity. The 1960s in the United States was a time of changing focus, including the Presidential Physical Fitness awards program early in the decade. The government had decided to push childhood fitness as a goal across the country. This, in a country where sport and sports heroes were already well established, brought formal recognition of physical development down to the elementary school level. The confluence of who I was "by nature" and the attributes my culture valued came together perfectly. Winning contests and being stronger and faster than your peers are rewarding outcomes for anyone at any age. Additionally, there were the social rewards from peers and adults that were separate and more long-lasting and pervasive than the powerful, but more immediate, effect of the direct rewards; good athletes in the US of A, are made to feel very special.

The years went by and because I continued to grow and develop ahead of schedule, by age 14 or so I had essentially grown to my full current height and had for the most part filled out across the shoulders and chest, which is to say I had the physical development of about a 22-year-old at an early age. I was beginning to enter local, then regional, then state and finally national competitions in a variety of sport. When one rises in level of competition or competence, it becomes clear that many of the attributes that may have been special at the local level become less so as one advances. The natural advantages of size, strength, and coordination became common among the competitors I was now encountering, and winning was no longer the easy, assured outcome it had been. I had always been a voracious reader and, as with my physical development, usually a little beyond where my cohorts were at any given time. My reading as it related to sport and physical development was usually about technique—how to throw the shot put farther, how to "clean and jerk" more weight, how to perfect the wrestling move, or how to receive the baton more smoothly to anchor the relay. The 1960s were also a time of social upheaval: new thoughts and ideas were entering the culture. Organic gardening and the notion of natural foods were not merely odd ideas that "hippies" were interested in—"healthy" began to take on new meaning. Eastern philosophies were becoming known and discussed not only in lonely mountain-top retreats but among secular groups as well. One effect of this milieu for me was a growing idea that it was not enough to have the strongest muscles, the fastest legs; how I cared for the body generally counted towards better performance on the field of sport. So it wasn't all just strength, speed, and technique: there were over-arching issues as well because general nutrition, the state of the stomach and the bowels at the time of competition, and being well rested and recuperated all had an impact on performance. As I read farther, it became clear that while it may not figure directly at the time of competition, the state of my organs affected the way my body performed. A healthy pulmonary system, liver, pancreas, and so on were brought to bear at the time of competition.

It was at about this time that I came across a book, *The Body Has a Head* by G. Eckstein (1970). It told the story of how the brain influences the body (the brain being the repository of the mind). What a concept! What and how you think may affect your body?! Western thought, culminating in Descartes, was all about *dualism*—the separation of mind (soul) and body. Western philosophies were becoming more accepting of Eastern philosophies (many of which did not make the mind/body distinction so strongly, or not at all), and Western medicine was beginning to explore the role the brain has on physical functioning. This then was the time within sport when people began to think about the effects "mental rehearsal," meditation, and other new concepts could have on performance, and I was no exception. I began learning about yoga and meditation, and to incorporate "mind-clearing" exercises before competing.

This was all very exciting and intellectually stimulating, and I began to read even more widely about Eastern and Western philosophies. The Indian philosopher, Jiddu Krishnamurti, was a huge influence on my thinking. Whenever I explore a topic, I like to look for commonalities, but how could the mind/body dualism of Western thought meld with the notion of the transience of the physical world in Eastern thought? In the simplest of terms, it is the notion of something bigger, more encompassing than the self—the connectedness of the individual to the whole. The whole community, the whole culture, the whole world, and, pushed to its limits, the whole universe of the known and the unknown. We tend to refer to the varying forms of these notions as *spirituality*.

So where does this lead us? While it is our cultural linguistic habit to speak of physical development and spiritual development as separate entities, they are in fact not. The leap that is made is the idea that they are two aspects of the same thing and, by nature, inseparable. You may be familiar with the story of Einstein's brain. Albert Einstein, one of the most famous mathematicians and geniuses of the 20th century died in 1957. His brain was removed and studied by brain scientists to discover what it was about his brain that made him so smart. After many years and many studies, the central finding was that Einstein's brain was in fact…essentially the same as everyone else's! The mistake was in believing that somehow the brain is the repository of who we are—but was not Einstein's liver as important to who Einstein was, as was his brain? Einstein could no more be Einstein without his liver than without his brain.

Later on and to this day as a psychologist and behavior analyst my broadest understanding of these phenomena is through the study of behavior. One way to conceptualize this is that we are what the whole body does and our *being* is an inseparable construct that flows from behaving in the world and being part of it. The analytical study of behavior has proved an efficient way to bring together the study of science and philosophy to inform practice—both my professional practice and my practice of becoming fully human. The coming together of mind and body presages, I believe, a coming together of spirituality and science in Western thought—again, two aspects of the same thing (see any of William Baum's writings on Buddhism and Behavior Analysis for more). Part of this is the understanding that the present moment is all there ever is and all there ever will be. Quoting my mentor, Howard Rachlin, in his book, *The Science of Self-Control* (2000, pp.3–4):

> The alcoholic does not choose to be an alcoholic. Instead he chooses to drink now, and now, and now, and now. The pattern of alcoholism emerges in his behavior (like saving [nuts] emerges in the behavior of the squirrel) without ever being chosen.

The same is true for all of our behavior, whether the outcome is for the good or the bad.

What Mr. Rubio has done with this volume is the beginning of bringing the mind and body together as one in a therapeutic way that is especially real and meaningful for people on the autism spectrum, particularly for teens and young adults with Asperger's Syndrome. He asks the correct question, I believe: "What do we have to *do* to begin achieving the union of brain and body?" He provides a philosophical underpinning and, even more importantly for the people he works with, a path of *doing* that leads to the achievement of goals well beyond the stated objectives. In a group of people so profoundly alone, as many with Asperger's Syndrome would tell you they are, Mr. Rubio introduces the idea of the *mentor*. Mentoring, while not new, has not been previously applied to this population in such a formal and philosophical way. The notion of *warriorship*, not the Western concept of male-dominated aggression, but rather as gender-neutral character development, is introduced as a meaningful archetype to explore behaving humanely to one's self, one's community, and the world at large; again the idea that there is something bigger, more fulfilling than merely the self.

I have set out a synopsis of my personal journey in hopes of reflecting the personal journey that each reader and each person touched by the concepts in this book will take. This book can be read and be useful as a set of techniques, but it is so much more engaging and meaningful as the beginning of a process to know yourself and the world.

Anthony Castrogiovanni, Ph.D.
Pyramid Educational Consultants (PECS) Olivebridge, NY

1

Introduction to Core Concepts of Pathfinder Mentoring

Three central concepts in my "Pathfinder" practice are: the holistic model upon which the training is based; the warrior archetype, an ideological concept that I've found to be an effective tool for mentoring; and the idea of rites of passage. The last of these, rites of passage, will be explored in the final chapter of this book. The first two will be explained here as an introduction to the fundamentals of my approach, a way of putting the practice of Pathfinder mentoring into context.

The holistic mind/body model in Pathfinder mentoring

The holistic model is the core vision upon which Pathfinder training is structured. The concept of holism (dealing with wholes, as opposed to parts of a whole) evokes images of the oneness of mind and body—of inner faith and honor of what is sacred. Warriorship (explored in more detail later in this chapter) is the teaching vehicle in Pathfinder training, and holism is the fuel that propels the individual to a place of deeper personal transformation.

Since ancient times, the martial arts and the warrior arts have been deeply intertwined with the religious or spiritual beliefs and thoughts of those times. This connection between the spiritual path and the warrior path helped develop the warrior's understanding that to live life fully is to fully execute one's commitments—one's mission—with calmness in spirit, mind, and body, no matter what adversity is faced. The knowledge that the warrior honors the sacredness of each moment, each breath, enables him to release the numbing, mind-killing effects of fear. For the warrior understands that life is in the moment and that one's inevitable death is held close to one's heart so as to release fear.

I practiced holism for self-survival. In 1979 as a young man living alone in New York City with little money for doctors and health insurance, I sought information to help me heal from my dance injuries and to create a program of preventative health measures. From books and treatments on acupressure, reflexology, homeopathy, Jin-Shin, massage, and nutritional concepts, I developed a way to take care of myself and help my dance friends as well.

I realized that the quality and effectiveness of my body healing was only as good as the quality of my mindfulness and my faith in my body's ability to heal. I went into the study of what was holy to me, what was sacred to me, of what was my faith system. This holistic mind/body training system that I developed in 1985 is called "*BodyKi*."

Early childhood and adolescent years were marked with physical and emotional abuse that left me with a sense of myself in fragments and pieces—fragile, ungrounded, and spacey, prone to depression and angry outbursts of intolerance towards others, locked in a time in my past. Thus, I realized that my mind and spirit required as much healing as my body, and that in fact that all three were inseparably connected.

By blending East and West or "alternative health" with "traditional health" in ideology, I created for myself, and later for my future clients, a holistic approach to reclaiming empowerment for myself, as I purified and cleansed my spirit, psyche, mind, and body of my past traumas.

In Pathfinder work with male mentees, aged 8–35 years old, the beginning of the training in warriorship is to know the meaning and honoring of what is holy and sacred in ourselves as individuals and, to a greater sense, as humans. I make it very clear to my mentees that I am talking about a sacred belief system that expresses our hearts and souls in a very deep and personal way.

Most of my 8–14-year-old clients with Asperger's Syndrome (AS) have a defined understanding of what religion is and usually practice a faith chosen by their parents. The 15–23-year-olds have a mixture of a personally evolved God or Great Spirit belief system with some remnants of past family religious practices, which they gave up and only practice when visiting home. Many of the older clients have a belief system that they have forgotten to honor and believe in and, therefore, live in a spiritual world of their making that is as illusive as fog.

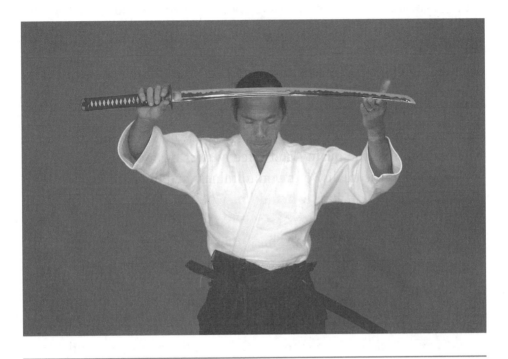

Sacred

The question I ask my clients is, "What is sacred and holy to you?" I offer no qualifications as to what is sacred and holy. I do offer examples:

> For instance, in some countries it is an animal that is deemed sacred such as the cow in India and the bald eagle here in America. There are special mountains and other powerful earth structures around the world that are regarded as holy and sacred. What is sacred and holy to you is a very personal and deeply meaningful object of your heart's attention.

When meeting a client for the first time, I conduct a standard information-gathering interview that gives me a basic picture of the current challenges being faced and their history. From there, I enter into the holistic approach that engages the client's whole being in a profound way. For in seeing and addressing the client as a holistic energetic being, I can re-vitalize or stimulate many levels of the client's own potential healing process. In building a relationship between two people, there is an essence in humans that is vibrantly charged with being fully aware and fully engaged in the totality of what is transpiring during the moments of inter-action. I aspire to this level of connection with all my clients.

From a holistic standpoint AS, autism spectrum disorder (ASD), attention deficit hyperactivity disorder (ADHD), pervasive developmental disorder (PDD), post-traumatic stress disordern (PTSD), obsessive com-pulsive disorder (OCD), and all the other "disorders" are only describing a part of the whole person. Although the distracting "meltdown" behaviors from the teen who has AS might be of great concern to teachers and parents, those behaviors are just a small part of the whole person.

That is the reason why I ask my students for information about their diet, their sleeping patterns, whether they bite their nails, and so on. What clues does their body language offer? What can I tell from the wear of their shoes, how they sit in a chair, how they stand, walk, and run? What language do they use to describe themselves and their lives? If I meet the divorced mother of an adolescent client, I would ask about the dynamics of the divorce and try to ascertain for how long before the break-up the child was exposed to any fighting, bickering, and so on. I ask about the birth and delivery of the client. This is some of the information I gather to "see" a holistic image of the client. I address the whole person as I purify the toxic fragments of their past that may be giving strength to their present-day challenges. It is the act of retrieving what was once whole from a place of pieces and chaos.

The "Clear vase" visualization exercise in Chapter 3 was developed early in my *BodyKi* practice to meet the need to offer a visual stimulation of wholeness through which to lead the client to consolidate mind/body awareness. I discovered that the "Clear vase" visualization exercise was effective with my clients who were rehabilitating from minor or major surgery, injury or trauma of any kind. Later in my Pathfinder mentoring, I intuitively implemented the "Clear vase" visualization exercise with my adolescent clients with AS as a playful exercise to remind them about their "whole self" and that from this place of wholeness they could address and change what they wanted to change as long as they involved their whole selves.

To conclude, I discovered in my Pathfinder mentoring, as well as in my *BodyKi* training, that the holistic paradigm opens great opportunities and new perspectives about personal transformation to be offered to the client/mentee, where in the past these opportunities and perspectives would have never been considered. This holistic training involves thinking "out of the box." It is exciting and calls forth the behaviors of perseverance, fortitude, and daring to challenge the norm. As Captain Kirk would say, "To boldly go where no man has gone before!"

The warrior and the hero archetype in Pathfinder mentoring: An interface to mentoring

Most of the males with AS with whom I have worked have had experiences playing with fantasy hero/warrior adventure strategy computer or video games. The gaming interests start at a young age with cartoons of popular hero characters and *Yugi-oh* game cards—moving up to the Dungeons and Dragons game and a multitude of fantasy, hero/warrior character, role-playing, video and computer games. It is with this pseudo hero/warrior background and interest much alive in their consciousness that I communicate the development and enhancement of a balanced warrior's energy and utilize the warrior's valuable life teachings. The client's game playing provides the perfect interface to where I begin my mentoring work.

With all my clients of any age, those with AS and those who are neuro-typical alike, I let it be known that in Pathfinder warriorship training the desired goal is to apply what is learned on the *dojo* mat or in a private session into one's daily life. Pathfinder mentoring emphasizes the utilization of the physical martial expression, as well as the teaching of the virtues that are contained within the physical training. These warrior/hero virtues promote an awareness of sacredness and the honoring of ourselves, as well as all living and non-living beings. Warrior virtues inspire perseverance, dedication to one's visions, stout inner discipline, and clear focus on achieving such intentions.

I have found the use of a holistic warriorship mentoring model to be an energetically dynamic approach in working with individuals who may have been adrift in the chaos of unwanted behaviors and detrimental

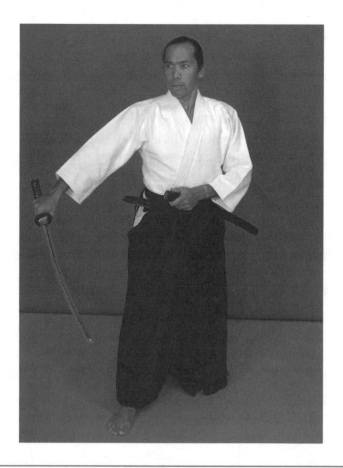

Warrior and hero

cognitive thinking processes, because it allows the individual with AS, who is so lacking in self-confidence and self-respect, to find the inner courage and spark to ignite the movement of personal revelations into action. This change starts from a place deep in their spiritual, emotional, and psychological core. For it is in the strengthening of the inner core of a person that I seek first to facilitate the possibility of a greater degree of success when working towards the completion of a set target goal.

The warrior is the defender and the fighter—the protector and one who serves the society. The warrior bleeds and sacrifices their own life without self-pity or regret. In the warrior heart there beats the drum of duty, discipline, and integrity of the self and unit: comrades in arms. Through the ages, the warrior has been a symbol of personal strength, honor, integrity, and a focussed discipline to a cause higher than the self.

There is a common belief that the warrior "is a masculine energy form" and, furthermore, this belief "persists because the warrior is a basic building block of masculine psychology, almost certainly rooted in our genes" (Moore and Gillette 1990). It is important to note, however, that the warrior since antiquity has been both male and female.

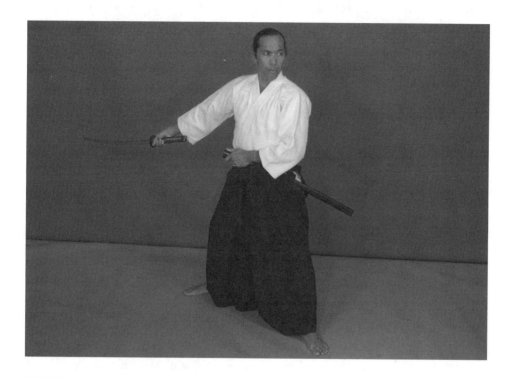

The warrior

When I introduce Pathfinder holistic warriorship to my mentees and students, I describe the polar expressions of the warrior energy. At one end of the scale is the "berserker warrior" and at the other end, to balance the berserker warrior, is the "healer warrior." And of course all the other expressions of the warrior are in between.

The berserker warrior expression has caused untold horror and destruction while defending "the cause." In the heat of battle, the berserker energy kicks in and the total destruction begins. In ancient times, warriors coming home from battle needed the entire village to bring the berserker warrior back to a safe place of warriorship where he would be able to once again walk among his community without "losing it." Modern wars have seen varying displays of the "welcome home" for their warriors from jubilant parades to being spat on and called "baby killers." Or the welcome home from World War II battlefronts that the Afro-American soldier received, which was to return to the discrimination laws that still prevailed in the south in the 1940s. The lack of community supported "decompression"—a show of appreciation for the validation and honoring of the warrior's sacrifices, efforts, and loss by their home community, and recognition of the necessity for the warrior to resume a normal life—some veteran warriors would stuff their anger and disappointments and experiences of loss deep inside themselves. The deadly bomb of unexpressed emotions and experiences would go off days, weeks, months, or many years later in self-destructive ways in which their families, their communities, and in the end the warriors themselves were the victims of the destruction.

The berserker warrior energy is important to understand and to utilize when under life-threatening situations where timing and utter destruction of the threat guarantees one's survival. The training in most martial arts is to know how to turn on the berserker energy, to control such energy when called upon and then to turn off the berserker energy and stand down when the situation is all clear. In the women's self-defense classes I teach, for example, the training speaks about this asset of being able to control, call forth, and unleash the berserker energy on a would-be rapist or attacker. It is incredible to witness a trained 4ft 5ins tall woman utterly devastate and destroy a fully padded would-be trainer "rapist" in a matter of seconds.

Balancing the berserker warrior energy is that of the healer warrior. The healer warrior energy is that of unconditional love and compassion for all on earth. The healer warrior is the navy corpsman attached to a marine platoon and risking their life for the medical care for their platoon mates, and at times those of the enemy. The healer warrior cares for the welfare of earth and cleans up oil spills and other man-made environmental disasters. The healer mends and heals those injured by the berserker. In ancient times, the warrior arts included the study of healing arts of reviving an opponent from injury or stabilizing a serious inflicted wound until other measures could be taken to preserve life.

The healer warrior identifies the life in battle and not death. This is not to say in the heat of battle a healer warrior would not protect the life of a comrade by taking the life of an enemy or adversary seeking to inflict injury. The healer warrior is still a warrior.

Often the hero energy is related to the warrior energy. The "hero" in our post-9/11 society brings forth such images that are of heart-wrenching displays of personal sacrifice to save another. The hero has traveled through the portals of ancient human to 21st-century homo sapiens' collective consciousness. The hero responds to dire situations without any regard to their own welfare. The hero presents an energy of being valiant, courageous without any question, and displaying an unwavering faith of completion of a seemingly impossible to task to be accomplished under extreme conditions in order to save lives. The hero in us is willing to fight for righting the injustice of others and standing ground against bullies and tyrants. The psychological and emotional charge of the hero in our cellular memory continues to be displayed in our cognitive and muscular behavior and actions when called upon to respond to someone else's distress and tragedy.

These two powerful archetypal energies, the warrior and the hero, can be welded into one entity, which can produce a deep-rooted positive shift in the mentality and behavioral aspects of young people if taught properly.

As a teacher of the martial arts I found that, when I utilized a warrior/hero mentality and the virtues of duty, discipline, and integrity in my teaching lessons with clients and students, the response was the creation of a positive teacher and student relationship founded in the virtues of honor, respect, mutual trust, and sincerity. In the martial arts, the teacher (*sensei*) embodies the warrior virtues that invoke the respect of the student's trust in their *sensei*'s leadership, knowledge, and martial mastery.

To this day, I remember with clarity and profound hindsight my time as a full-scholarship dance student and how I embraced the concepts and practice of inner discipline and focus by the honoring of the training of the senior teachers of the Alvin Ailey School of Dance. The teachers instilled an honoring of personal power and presence that spoke of a personal conviction of empowerment without fear. These are similar to characteristics found as a product of in-depth martial art training.

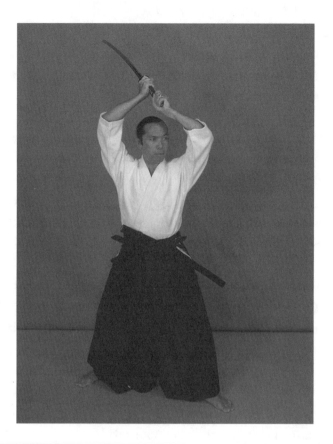

Teacher of martial arts

When, as teachers, we ask our students to follow us—to obey our word—we are asking them to trust our judgment and wisdom. Quality leadership in warriorship is a vital cog in the wheel in building a sound working relationship. When working with ASD individuals, I always make it a point to inform my new clients at the beginning of the session that "I am not perfect and I do not know everything. Yet, I know enough to be teaching you correctly and effectively. I am looking forward to enjoying our working relationship." I also tell them, " I won't waste your time if you won't waste my time. I am not here to nag or whine or baby-sit. I am here to mentor, teach, guide and help you. I won't let you down or leave you behind. In return your best efforts are expected by me."

That little pep talk works wonders because, through my body language and the sincerity in my voice, and by my actions and behavior, the students and mentees learn to know and trust that I mean what I say and I am as good as my word—very positive warrior leadership traits to teach and communicate.

I walk a hero's path for my clients to see. This path of proper manners, etiquette, respect for others, and a positive display of personal empowerment requires me to be fair and honest about myself. Exposing my own past failings and disasters through teaching stories with my mentees enables me to call their bluffs and challenge their disruptive behaviors safely and with an authority that is honored and respected. This mentoring path requires me to go the distance with them and to go out on a limb for them. I walk this path in return for their honesty, sincerity, and their focussed attention on our work together and on their personal lives.

As a hero and a warrior mentor, I know when to act boldly and push a student's comfort zone, and when to show patience and compassion when their "growing pains" are too much for they themselves to handle. In a charged moment in a classroom where a meltdown is brewing with an AS student, I know when to stand my ground or strategically retreat, although it might be uncomfortable for all involved, so as to resolve the crisis safely. The action of "strategic retreat" is implemented in order to regroup and ground myself with the AS student, and therefore create an opening—a pause and space to allow the unseen and un-thought of options to materialize and be utilized for a positive outcome.

As a Pathfinder mentor, the warrior and the hero archetypes and the emotional and physical energies of the warrior and hero that resonate from within the client's own psyche—from a deeply embedded experience in the collected human consciousness—are exciting and awe-inspiring to use. When used properly, the warrior and the hero strengthen the faith and visions of the mentee as they continue to evolve and mature.

Effects of the warrior archetype in practice

With most of my teenaged clients with AS, I have experienced hard jarring times and struggles in their behavioral evolution that appear like "speed bumps" in the process of releasing persistent and deeply entrenched detrimental thinking, such as intolerance to change something about themselves in order to reach a desired goal. Here is an example of how, using the archetypal warriorship to influence and promote a difficult transformation.

Something that is often hard for mentees with AS is getting out of the safe comfort zone of wearing their comfortable baggy sweat or exercise pants and the too large tee shirt or sweatshirt that they are so used to, and accepting the fact that they must wear other more acceptable attire to a job interview. For some of my clients with AS, to think of wearing anything but their clothing of choice is ludicrous and outright impossible even to imagine, let alone actually do.

So, when a particular mentee was speaking to me about the reality of his maturing desires and wants, his initial outlook was: "I want a GameCube and new games and my parents do not have or will not give me the money for it." I said to my mentee:

> Maybe you need a job to make money to get those items. So you have to look sharp for a job interview in order to get even a crack at the job opportunity—first impressions are important—and if you want it badly enough you have to go after it and do whatever it takes to achieve this goal.

At this point I receive a major—"You are out of your mind and you must be crazy"—look from the mentee. I continue:

> So you have to be courageous and extremely focussed and disciplined to accomplish this goal to get work. It will take a great willingness to change something you feel so strongly about, yet you know it is something that is holding you back.

Then I remind the mentee of our warriorship training time together. At this time I had worked with this mentee for three years starting when he was 13.

> Remember what you have accomplished for yourself since you started the work with me and the warriorship training you have learned. You are a different person now than you were before. You have developed a discipline and focus that allows you to maintain clarity in your mind and stay grounded in your emotions and energy while you are under stress. You have come to terms with your past behaviors that you were so ashamed and frustrated about. You are different and no longer a little boy but a

young man now. Apply the warrior traits you are trained into now to challenge and persevere through this next level of your life.

Yes, it will be hard to wear the clothing you need to wear for a job interview. Yes, it might be uncomfortable to wear clothes you are not used to at first. And no, wearing these work clothes does not mean you are giving up something of who you are. See it as a costume you must wear to do a job and that is all. Most importantly, remember you can change anything you want in your life now for you understand how precious your life is—how sacred each moment of your life is. And most importantly, holding on to your past behaviors and comfort zones will not give the financial base to get what you want in your life today.

It came as no surprise that the AS mentee took a long hard look and realized that the truth was in his face. Slowly he started to change and become more receptive to the notion of wearing the appropriate clothes to go to a job interview.

It took great courage and insight for him to see the challenge, acknowledge the challenge, and then do something about it, rather than fight and scream about his old fears and let it go at that and never change.

The "Eye of the hurricane": Staying calm and centered under fire

In warriorship training, there is much discussion and study on how to stay calm under fire—how to reduce the factors of fear in order to survive. I call this concept in Pathfinder training the "Eye of the hurricane."

In some parts of the United States, the hurricane season is a very real and dangerous time of the year. Hurricanes pack a lot of energy that is built up by high winds and a mixture of hot and cold air. A hurricane can really wallop an area and lay waste to anything that stands in its path.

The power generated on the outside of these cone-shaped displays of elemental forces are high winds, torrential rain, and total mayhem. Contrary to its chaotic perimeter, the hurricane's "eye" or "center" is calm and stable. A paradox of energies existing in the same place at the same time with this dynamic relationship of opposites all contained into one entity—that is the hurricane.

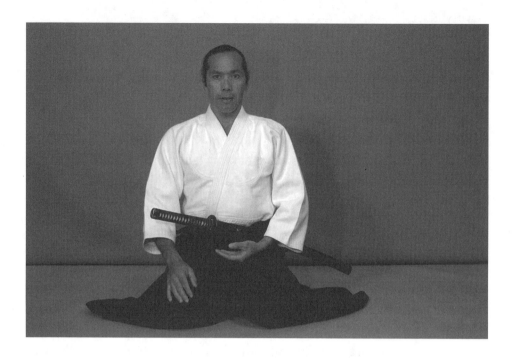

Eye of the hurricane

As I was starting my martial art training in *aikido*, I was already deeply involved in a professional dance career in New York City. One of the first things I noticed about this Japanese martial art was its powerful movements. Being a dancer, I was drawn to the circular movements found in most of the *aikido* techniques. I was amazed how an *aikidoka* (one who practices *aikido*) would be moving around a stable centerline of balance, while the partner or attacker would be sent flying like a leaf in the wind! It reminded me of hurricanes. As I continued to practice *aikido*, I was amazed to find myself calm and confident for, by using the centrifugal force of the *aikido* movement, my partner would be projected effortlessly away with fluid power.

I started to use this *aikido* technique as a conceptual affirmation right before a big dance performance because I would find myself very anxious immediately before going on stage. The affirmation was "Stay in the 'Eye of the hurricane.' Stay calm and stable." I would visualize myself dancing from a grounded emotional center and becoming a hurricane of choreographed movement and expression. The affirmation worked to center my focus and release anxiety and fear. My performances were flawless, executed with confidence and expressed with ease and power.

One way to calm and focus the mind is to focus on breathing in the present moment. From this focussed place, we can clearly see ourselves being in the "Eye of the hurricane."

When I first told my ASD and AS students about the "Eye of the hurricane," they loved the story and what it meant. Some really understood the "coolness" of being that stable and calm, while all around you things could be as crazy as a sinking ship.

Some of the young men in the class saw the connection to the story I had told them about the two dueling *samurais* and the intensity of the moment. They understood the importance of the mindful focus the two warriors needed to have in order to stay calm under such extreme stress. A lesson learned!

Another way to put this concept in to words is by a teaching poem that Morihei Ueshiba "O'Sensei" the creator of the Japanese martial art *aikido*, offered his students (Stevens 1992):

> Move like a beam of light;
> Fly like lighting
> Strike like thunder
> Whirl in circles around
> A stable center.

When we stand in front of an individual with AS having a meltdown because he has been introduced to an unforeseen change in his daily class schedule, we confidently stand on our own two feet, grounded in our posture and in the "Eye of the hurricane." We are prepared for the chaotic emotional stress and anxiety that he will express, and will support him back to earth and calmness.

When doing the mind/body exercises in this book, it is an excellent practice to "take the time to clear the slate" and "ground yourself" using *misogi* breathing before starting a class. This is explained fully in the following chapter. Before you take over a situation or jump into a hot one, take three deep breaths in a way that you can focus on your breathing. For even in those three breath cycles you will have created time for you to awake a sense of calmness and confidence with which to ground yourself.

Those three breaths will allow you time to focus your emotions, charge your physical awareness, and ignite your commitment to the moment at hand so that you can be 100 percent present. You are now centered and clear.

See in your mind's eye the stressful and chaotic energy on the periphery of your calmness, as you are the stable center. From this place of calmness and confidence in your skills and abilities, you can be the witness of the situation, size it up, and act promptly and effectively. In this way, you can remedy the crisis with direction, integrity, and compassion.

Breathe into the "Eye of the hurricane"—into your calmness and stability. Being in the "Eye of the hurricane" is the mark of a strong and sincere leader. From your "calmness under fire" your students will see that everything is ok and that everything has a solution and an ending. Your steadfastness will inspire the same in your students. They will understand that calmness and focus are beneficial behaviors that they can develop in themselves.

Notes on the *sempai–kohai* relationship:
A martial art relationship of trust

The relationship between *sempai* (*sem-pie*), meaning senior, and *kohai* (*ko-hi*), meaning junior, is a component of the martial arts I find effective when I am teaching and mentoring large groups. This relationship, with its beginnings in warriorship training can develop a communication of trust, respect, responsibility, reliability, and leadership between *sempai* and *kohai*.

When I first started *aikido* almost 23 years ago, I was introduced to this *sempai* and *kohai* relationship. I have *sempais* who have been my teachers and mentors in *aikido* for the 23 years I have been practicing. Some of my *sempais* are now my dear friends and considered part of my family. A deep sense of trust and respect exists between us.

I always knew I would be put in my place by my *sempai* if I was out of order. If I had a question about *aikido* techniques, protocol or anything relating to *aikido*, I would never hesitate to go to my *sempais* for guidance and support. In some cases I have not hesitated to call upon my *sempais* on issues outside of *aikido*.

Not all *sempais* were, to me, good *sempais*. Anyone of higher rank than me is my *sempai*. Yet, it was the quality of their character, their leadership, and compassionate guidance that signified them as true *sempais* to me. Nevertheless, a *sempai* is a *sempai* and respect is generally applied and expected from the *kohai*.

The first concept I introduce with my students is the *sempai–kohai* relationship. In a classroom environment, the *sempai–kohai* relationship is built around the students' ages. The first thing is defining who the *sempais* and *kohais* are. The 10–12-year-old "boys" are designated as the *kohais*, and the 13 years and older "young men" are the *sempais*. This first *sempai* and *kohai* grouping relates to the idea of Rites of Passage—the difference between boys and young men. These *kohai* and *sempai* groups are each subdivided into two groups. So within the first *kohai* group there is a *sempai* and *kohai* relationship and in the first *sempai* group there is a *sempai* and *kohai* relationship. What is developed is a hierarchy of the ages among the students, which allows me to develop age-appropriate behavior from them.

It is valuable for the older students, who are designated as the *sempais* of the class, to be made aware of aspects of their behavior that are deemed inappropriate for their ages. Acknowledging and validating their age, that they are now young men and not young boys, I believe, opens their eyes and minds to the potential of their present moment lives. It is like a splash of cold water on their faces—the reality of their inappropriate behavior and how it must look to others.

When in place and properly activated, the *sempai–kohai* model will develop the following virtues as mentioned previously:

- trust

- respect

- responsibility

- leadership

- reliability.

These virtues are interwoven and grow organically from each individual student to the entire class. You are the teacher, the mentor, and the

Pathfinder model of the virtues listed. When your students see you display these virtues honestly and sincerely, they will follow your lead.

You begin slowly to challenge the *sempais* of the class to stretch and grow. You offer your *sempais* responsibility within the class so they may develop positive leadership skills. The *sempais* are called upon to demonstrate any teachings you feel they can explain, show, or execute with confidence and empowerment. You build them up through teaching, mentoring, and guiding.

The *kohais* will learn by observing you, their primary teacher (*sensei*), while keeping both eyes on how their sempais respond and treat you. And if you mentor your sempais in this matter, you will see them shine by helping you out, which is an acknowledgment of their role as a sempai.

In time, the *kohais* in your group will in turn become *sempais* in their own right. And the circle continues and the class evolves as a community of individuals growing together. It is hard work and needs insightful planning on your part as their Pathfinder to keep the group dynamic growing and stretching outside their comfort zones. Like a tribe or family, this *sempai* and *kohai* relationship will experience the real-life dynamics from the painful and challenging growing pains to glorious life-enhancing revelations in behavior and in maturity.

Your leadership will weigh heavily in the success of the *sempai* and *kohai* relationship. Rely on your creativity, ingenuity, and improvisation to nurture this working relationship to full maturity and effectiveness.

2

The Breath Foundation: Being Grounded

We do not breathe in the past—We do not live in the past.
We do not breathe in the future—We are not living tomorrow.
We only breathe in the present moment—one breath at a time.
Change what you want to change of yourself right now.
Not in the past, not in the future.
Right now!
—With boldness and confidence.

(Pathfinder teaching poem)

A Pathfinder mentoring training session begins with the study of breath awareness—how you are breathing and how you are feeling in the moment. As the mentee breathes, talks, and moves, note is taken of their motor skills, balance, and coordination. Most importantly, I am evaluating their ability to breathe with ease, intention, and confidence in every movement and in every moment. The quality of the mentee's awareness in the moment is indicative of the evolution of the individual with autistic spectrum disorder (ASD) in every aspect of their lives. In the first session, it is also explained that making any changes in one's life, such as releasing an old detrimental behavior, is a process of taking and claiming small, sure steps of success, which build up until one can run with empowerment—built upon self-confidence, knowledge, and skill. So many times in the past the mentee was pushed to accomplish more than they could or given a goal that was unattainable. Small, sure steps produce big gains in developing confidence and personal faith.

While introducing breath awareness at the beginning of the mentor/mentee relationship, I also begin to "anchor" or "fix into place" whatever my teaching or mentoring goals are for the mentee into their minds and bodies through their breathing. Rather than simply verbalizing goals sitting down, anchoring goals while the mentee is actively breathing is like pouring information directly into their muscle cells, building new pathways in the brain. This form of anchoring information in the breath, mind, and body while mentoring, allows the mentee to process the information through each and every learning pathway possible.

Once learned, breath awareness can be used in small group situations as well. I once observed a classroom of autistic students and their teacher engage in five minutes of simple movement games, stretching and breathing exercises that I had previously taught them. These five minutes allowed everyone to take a break, settle down, and release tension and anxiety. When it was time to continue the class, the students were able to flow with the teacher more easily. The previous "on the edge meltdown" energy of the class was safely and energetically discharged. The exercises grounded everyone back down to earth to be recharged—a transmutation of energy. I could actually see and feel the change—the students' shoulders were relaxed and their minds focussed to the best of their abilities. At this point the teacher was teaching and the students were learning.

In my mentoring practice, I offer my mentees and myself this simple direction: "Breath will focus and calm my mind, and from a focussed and calm mind I focus my Body."

Through breath awareness, you have the grounded focus to change behavior and detrimental thought patterns; you can heal your body from injury and trauma; you can change your life to express the full potential of your existence.

Fundamental breathing exercises

A breath cycle = one (1) inhale + one (1) exhale = one breath cycle

In teaching exercises, I use a breath cycle count rather than a number count. So, for instance, it would be "do 20 breath cycles of sit-ups" rather than "give me 20 sit-ups."

Let's begin.

Instructor's note: If leading this exercise, the following is to be read out loud:

1. Please sit comfortably and try this—ok. Start by being aware of how you are breathing right now.

2. Good. Now let's try breathing in through the nose slowly (Figures 2.1, 2.2)…good! …and now slowly breathe out through your mouth very gently (Figure 2.3).

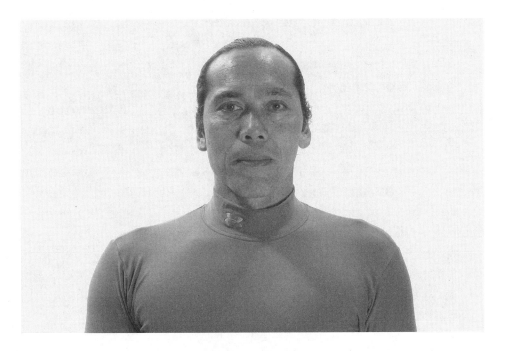

Figure 2.1 Relaxed face on the inhale through the nose

3. Great! Keep breathing in this manner: breathing in through your nose slowly…good…and breathing out of your mouth slowly…very good.

4. Here is a suggestion: try to keep your facial mask (your facial muscles) relaxed. Please try to release the need to form the letter "O" with your mouth or shape the lips when exhaling out of the mouth (Figures 2.4, 2.5).

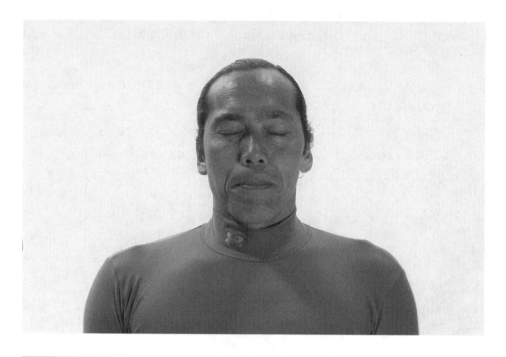

Figure 2.2 Incorrect: Closing eyes and losing connection on the inhale

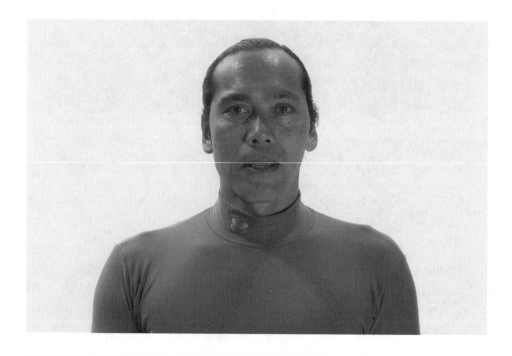

Figure 2.3 Relaxed face on the exhale out of the mouth

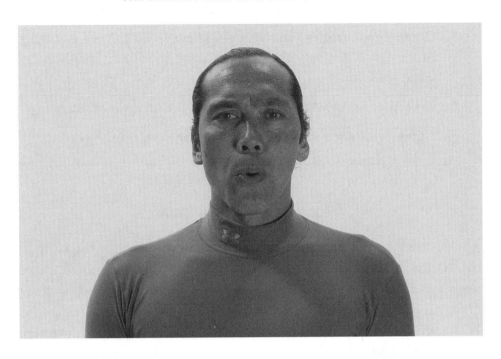

Figure 2.4 Incorrect: Exhaling out of the mouth with too much force

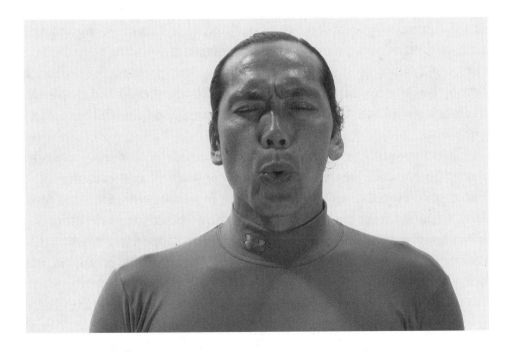

Figure 2.5 Incorrect: Too much force on the exhale with eyes closed

5. Great! Keep breathing this way. And now, while you are breathing, explore how you can relax your neck and shoulders. Try it and just take your time.

6. Great! Let's slowly finish. Let's do three breath cycles to finish.

7. Good. Breathing is natural and can be done in a relaxed way.

———————

Breathing with your belly

The next step is to explore how to send the breath cycle into the belly. In the martial arts, breathing in this fashion is described as breathing into one's center. Movement in the human body is most stable when one's gravity is centered in a lower part of the body, especially the pelvic girdle. With gravity low in the body, it is easier to accomplish dynamic movement and balancing. For example, a dancer can balance or spin on half point or full point, with confidence and ease, when the movement comes from a strong center of gravity and is guided by the breath.

I suggest to students who have a hard time understanding this concept of belly breathing to observe the breathing of babies or young animals such as kittens and puppies. Infant mammals breathe in their bellies, showing a sense of safety and relaxation. Fear, traumatic experiences, tension and stresses can drive the breath cycle into our chest and shoulders. This makes our shoulders and neck muscles tired and achy, and may affect our mood.

I used to suffer from severe asthma. I was all "shoulders—no neck" during an asthmatic attack. It was frightening as well as exhausting to be fighting for every breath, because this was in a time before inhalers. Years later, I learned from my martial training how to use breathing from my lower body and dropping my center of gravity to support movement. I discovered that breathing from my lower body freed up my shoulders and neck.

In belly breathing our lungs will fill and empty naturally. Belly breathing allows for a deeper sense of breath and a deeper sense of core strength and self-awareness. Belly breathing also allows our earthly gravity to settle in the most stable area of our bodies: the pelvic girdle.

Belly breathing exercise

Instructor's note: If leading this exercise, the following is to be read out loud:

1. This is an exercise in breathing more with your belly, or stomach area, rather than with your upper body—upper chest, shoulders, and neck.

2. Please sit upright in your chair. (This is best done lying on the floor if space is available.) Thank you. Now, please place your hands over your belly or stomach area. Place your left hand first on your belly area and then your right hand over the left hand.

3. Let's begin our breathing like we learned before. That's right: breathing in through your nose slowly…good! …and now slowly breathing out of your mouth very gently. Great! Please continue breathing as I talk.

4. Now everyone try this: on your inhale through your nose, slowly fill or inflate your stomach like a balloon (Figure 2.6). Gently. That's right.

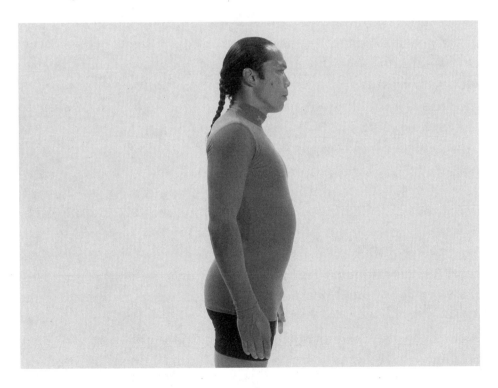

Figure 2.6 While you are inhaling, fill your belly like a balloon

5. Hold the inhale breath for a second and allow the breath to settle into the belly a little bit more. Good.

6. Now, as you exhale out of a relaxed mouth, gently flatten out your belly (Figure 2.7), exhaling all the breath out—completely out. Very nice everyone!

7. Remember, it is ok if you are challenged by this. It takes time to learn.

8. Continue to practice breathing in this manner, and just calmly notice at this time if your shoulders are relaxed on the inhale breath cycle. Do your shoulders raise up when you breathe in? They will rise gently without so much energy charge if you are focussing on breathing with your belly.

9. Focus calmly on releasing the shoulders, neck and face when you are breathing in. I know this may be challenging, yet it gets easier with practice I assure you.

10. Good try everyone!

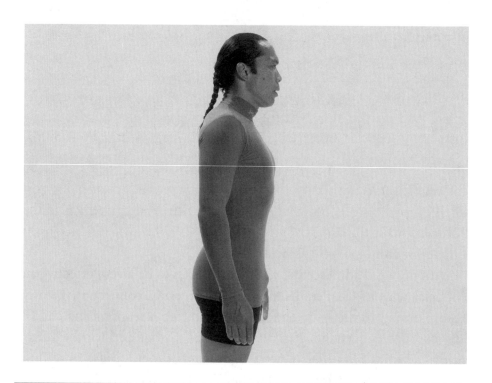

Figure 2.7 While exhaling out of your mouth, flatten and deflate your belly

Clearing the slate: Emptying the cup
Misogi: Breathing concept and exercises

When I work with my clients or students, one of the concepts I explain while introducing breathing exercises is *misogi*. *Misogi* is a Japanese term, which means "to purify or to cleanse."

Most martial art training includes a spiritual component. Words such as sacred, holy, or purification can be expressed in a holistic manner in either the study of warriorship or spirituality—an illustration of the balance of the archetypal energies of the warrior and the healer (faith). So, when developing breathing awareness with students through exercises, I use language and stories to evoke a sense of the preciousness of the present moment. Such as the following:

> Long ago in medieval Japan two members of the *samurai* class prepared to duel on a dry open plain. Their *katanas*, their killing swords, were drawn.
>
> The day was still and a cloudless sky draped above them. It seemed that the very life around the two warriors stood quiet and still—waiting for the ensuing action to occur. Once the *katanas* were drawn, honor and discipline forbade the sheathing of them: life or death was the only path of action to follow.
>
> They stood, seemingly forgotten by the world around them, where time is a precious and sacred moment that could never be taken back or relived, when suddenly one moved in a flash and the other responded in like. And within a heartbeat and a flutter of eyelids one *samurai* remained standing and the other lay mortally wounded, dying. (A Pathfinder teaching story)

This warrior story illustrates for the students the concept of being completely present in every moment. The importance of being aware of oneself in order to make the right choices in life speaks of how sacred each breath in the present moment—the now—really is.

With my ASD adolescents, *misogi* has proven to be a very effective and beneficial way to clear and unite the mind/body connection before a session, during challenging times and closing up a session. The child or teen may not understand it at first. And yes, I often receive the "this is boring" attitude from the students the first time we do *misogi* breathing exercises. However, after a while, they learn to like and appreciate the calming and focussing benefits. They learn that breathing exercises create a moment of pause—a sacred moment to reorganize the focus; to very slowly come back to earth from a meltdown; or to just take the moment to prepare for a transition. Learning to regroup and get centered before transitions is very useful for those with autism, and for anyone who gets anxious about moving on to the next activity or trying something new.

We can see *misogi* then as a way of "clearing the slate or emptying your cup." This practice allows the student to surrender preconceived ideas of themselves and make room for present moment changes. This is a very important concept for any adolescent, ASD and neuro-typical student alike, who is discouraged from years of "being behind the eight ball." A history of bad experiences can result in a toxic level of low-self esteem—triggered when under stress and anxiety. Internal chatter starts playing over and over like a broken record in the student's mind, such as "I can never succeed because I failed in the past at doing this (or something) like this." Spiritually, mentally, physically, and emotionally, the student will unconsciously or consciously sabotage any effort towards success. Their negative anchors fire up and are expressed in any combination of disruptive, resisting behavior, such as fooling around and provoking others around them to act out. Or the student will just shut down and not try it at all. Period. A common teacher error is to label the student as oppositional or difficult. This results in a power struggle, which only causes the insecure student to dig their heels in more deeply. An experienced mentor, teacher, or therapist will recognize and address the underlying anxiety.

In order to change a detrimental behavior effectively, one needs to empty the space inside one's mind and heart that is clinging to memories of past failures. Clearing this space makes room for new ideas and behavior to be suggested, tried, and implemented in the present moment of the now. Feeling comfortable and at ease from breathing awareness helps a lot while going through challenging times at home, school, or in a job.

In martial training, as in chemistry and biology, a basic premise holds true: voids that are created are immediately filled. A martial art example would be dodging a punch and using the opening to execute a counter punch: filling the void—decisively and boldly. This can easily be applied to the mentoring and teaching of challenging individuals. While in the process of *misogi* with a student, decisively and with great wisdom, fill the space of the vacancy left by eliminating the targeted detrimental behavior in the student's consciousness with the teachings of positive life-transforming mentorship. As those engaged in the process of change understand, one does not give up old patterns of behavior until new ones are available and accepted.

The following *misogi* breathing exercise is done with a simple body movement. However, *misogi* breathing can also be the simple act of sitting quietly and breathing with attention to the quality of calmness. The student can adjust the use of *misogi* to the situation. For example, if a student has a movement break or free time, they can utilize the movement sequence as well as the breath. If the student is in a social situation such as a class lecture, movement might be inappropriate. In that case, they can still calm and focus themselves through the intention of their breath without disturbing others. As I have explained to my students through the years, "*Misogi* is a breath to breath phenomenon. The gesture of *misogi* need not be dressed with anything but sincerity and truth."

Once the mentee understands *misogi* movement, and their breath rhythm settles into a seamless current of focussed, calm attention, I bring visualization into play. I add visualization to enhance the effects of *misogi*. Visualization is the practice of seeing an image in one's mind. Sometimes I describe it as seeing "In the mind's eye."

The white light visualization

I use white light because of its neutralizing quality. As with white paint, white light allows for the dilution of any other color back towards white. Thus, white light suggests a purifying quality to dissipate and dislodge past detrimental energy from its hold upon the student's consciousness and perception of themselves. *Misogi* breathing along with white light visualization helps remove obstacles in the way of their positive growth forward.

Visualization exercises are to be applied with a sense of creativity, playfulness, and innovation offered in an environment free from judgmental views of a "right" or "wrong" way. The participant will adapt at their own pace with their own interpretations. The mentor guides with a great sense of tolerance and acceptance: adjust your technique for the participant. For example, David, one of my mentees with Asperger's Syndrome (AS), reported that he was completely unable to visualize. What David could do well was to describe his inner experience kinesthetically, using words that described the quality of the emotional and physical sensations he was experiencing. Instead of asking David to visualize white light (which would have caused him to resist and shut down), we developed a language specifically for him: "David, as you practice *misogi*, allow the tight tense rock in your stomach to become softer and softer, crumbling away a little at a time with each breath. Can you *feel* that David? Great!" (instead of saying, "Can you see or imagine that, David?").

Misogi with body movement exercise

Instructor's note: If leading this exercise, the following is to be read out loud:

1. Before starting, please choose a particular challenge that you are facing and that you wish to clear the slate of/get rid of. For example, maybe you are worried about your homework, or scared that you won't be good enough at doing something, like learning how to drive.

2. Now, please stand. Stand firmly now (Figure 2.8) and let's begin.

3. This is a breathing exercise called *misogi*. It is to help you clear your mind and settle down should you feel stress and anxiety building up because you are nervous or an old fear has reared up. *Misogi* means to purify or to cleanse. It is a Japanese word. In the martial arts, the *misogi* breathing exercise is used to focus and prepare one's mind and body.

4. Start your breathing cycle like you have learned previously, in through your nose and out through the mouth. Now on your inhale cycle, raise your arms up your sides with palms facing upwards until your fingertips touch above your head (Figures 2.9, 2.10, 2.11). Great! (or let us try that again).

5. Hold here for a moment as you sink your breath into your belly, and on your exhale breath cycle slowly allow your hands to float down the front and center of your body with your fingertips touching (Figures 2.12, 2.13). Great!

6. This movement is repeated with your breath cycle. The timing of the movement is timed with the rhythm of your breathing.

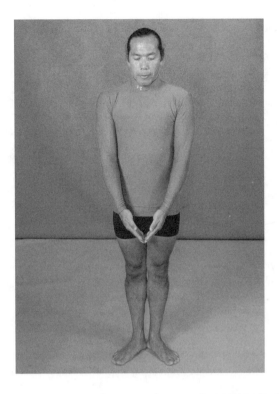

Figure 2.8 Starting position—neutral

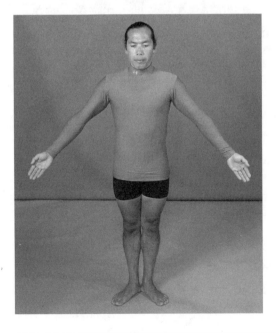

Figure 2.9 Begin to raise your hands and head slowly as you inhale through your nose

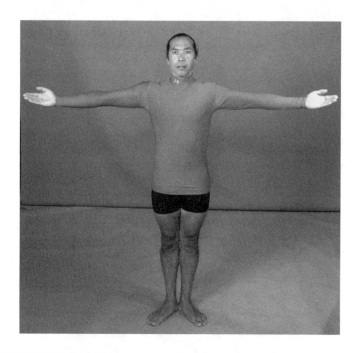

Figure 2.10 Keep shoulders down as arms move towards zenith above head

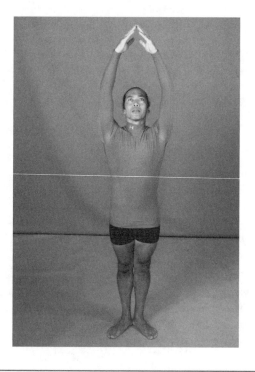

Figure 2.11 Hold arms at zenith and gently hold breath

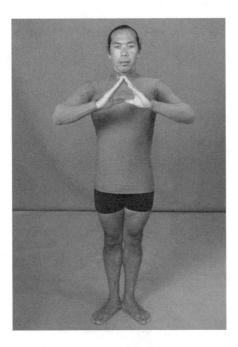

Figure 2.12 Slowly begin to lower arms and head on the exhale down the middle line of your body

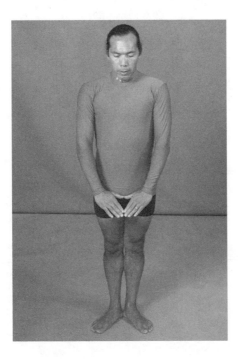

Figure 2.13 Continue to exhale gently out of your mouth as your head and arms descend down the middle line of your body…and finish back at neutral

7. You move in concert with your breathing. Your breath is the meter, the timing, for your movement.

8. Begin the visualization of white light entering your whole self. In your inhale cycle and with your exhale cycle, use the white light to flush out the challenge you have chosen to work on today. Good, keep it up.

9. Allow your breathing with the white light to dissolve and wipe clean the old patterns of the challenge you are working on.

10. Clearly see the inhale breath in the form of white light.

11. Clearly see the exhale breath in the form of white light.

12. Allow your breath to "sweep the slate clean": to normalize your energy flow through your entire self.

————————

3

Mindfulness:
Taming "the Chattering Mind"

Students with autism spectrum disorder (ASD) are challenged with a neurological disability that affects their ability to grow and mature cognitively, emotionally, behaviorally, and physically. Their mindfulness, their ability to be aware of what is going on around them—during the process of learning new behaviors—is vital. The ASD student will discover that their pro-active contribution to the process of change, when they are mindful of the present moment, will empower them with a sense of intention.

In some martial arts disciplines, there is a name for "mindlessness"—it is called "the chattering mind." The chattering mind is like having a "monkey on your back." To an ASD individual, this one monkey can feel like a whole troop of monkeys!

Should this inner dialogue, this "chattering mind" ramble unchecked in our heads, we might find ourselves detached from the present moment and from what is happening right now, or we might find ourselves acting out based upon the garbled inner dialogue. It is no wonder we sometimes lock ourselves out of our house or car. Or maybe we fire off at what we misperceived someone had said, rather than really listening to what is truly being communicated.

The chattering mind is the inner dialogue in our minds. This inner dialogue draws from a vast library of information from our personal experiences, fantasies, and other memories. When the common daydreamer accesses this huge store of information, they drift off to a very different, and sometimes vividly experienced, place from the one they are physically in at the moment. I am sure that, if you are a teacher, parent, or caregiver, you have observed the ASD student "disappear" to that place of distraction because of the stress and anxiety they experience when faced with certain tasks or situations. For some of the ASD males I have worked with, the place they go is the very engaging fantasy world of their video, playing card or computer games of sword and sorcery.

Memories are generated from experiences that a person has lived. Memories are charged into the body as a whole energetic charge—a breath, mind, and body experience. These memories are played out in our minds like movies when activated by a physical stimulation such as a certain smell, a similar sight, a particular sound, music, the weather, or even the heat or coolness in the room.

An individual can start feeling certain emotions that may have no relevance to the present moment experience. For instance, a client of mine was projecting her ideas of how she imagined the rehabilitation of a recent injury would unfold based on a similar injury she had experienced in her past. I introduced the facts that the circumstances of the current injury were different from that of her past injury: she was in very different physical shape now than she was then (she had lost 35 lbs), and she was using a very different method of rehabilitation this time around. The memory of the past injury had stimulated the emotions of fear, apprehension, anxiety, and self-defeat before we could even start working together.

In another example, a student with Asperger's Syndrome (AS) whom I was teaching refused to try a balancing movement that I was asking him to do along with his peers—other AS students. When I asked him why he did not want to even try the movement, he responded, "When I tried something similar to what you are asking me three years ago, I could not do it and everyone in my class laughed at me." Whoa. When I replied that he was three years older now (15 years old) and that I do not allow any student to laugh or ridicule another student's trying and not succeeding, he looked astounded and gave it a shot. Although he faltered at the first attempt, when he saw no one laughing or even looking funny at him, he tried again and again until he accomplished the movement. I shook his hand and he smiled.

I reminded him that our minds grow in a similar fashion to that of a baby learning to walk. First, we crawl, then we pull ourselves up to sitting, then to standing with support, and finally we let go of that support to take those first awkward steps. When we fall down, we get up and try again. I explained to this student that it takes great patience, perseverance, and discipline to stay in the process of change until your mind gets used to new ideas and behaviors that will allow you to transform into the "new and improved self!" The student liked that idea. The new and improved self!

His success pivoted on my support and the fact that I had addressed and successfully quietened down his chattering mind, which had triggered memories of past humiliation. We were able to get down to work and change. It is important to note that one of the most common forms that obsessive thinking takes for those with AS and other spectrum disorders is the focus on past failure, self-criticism, fears of making mistakes, and being criticized by others (Attwood 2006). Thus, uncovering and addressing these fears allows the student to move ahead in the present moment.

There is a place in our mind that is quiet and undisturbed from the internal chatter of past fears, self-doubts, frustration, self-directed anger, pain, or reliving the ecstasy of a past victory. When aware of the present moment and detached from the chattering, we can be effective in our lives. In the martial arts, there is a place in the beginning of class where you start with meditation breathing exercises, preparing the mind/body for training by clearing the slate—going to a place of quietness in spirit and mind.

It is better to simply observe the chattering mind rather than engage in dialogue with it. We are in a powerful state of awareness when the mind and body are settled, clear and ready to take on whatever challenge we are facing from a place of grounded calmness.

One of the goals I suggest to all my students and mentees is to try to be as mindful and aware as they possibly can, in every situation they are in. Mindfulness improves the quality of our interactions with ourselves and others, whether the task be learning social skills, movement, problem solving, or driving a car. The more mindful we are, the more connected, receptive, and responsive we are with ourselves, others, and our experience of life itself.

"Clearing the mind space" visualization

This is a basic visualization I use at the start of working with any new client. The "Clearing the mind space" visualization creates a neutral mind space—detachment from the inner chattering voices and distracting visions. Clearing the mind creates space for new information free from doubt, fear, pre-judgments, and self-criticism from the past.

Instructor's notes:

- Begin by doing a series of breath *misogi* exercises as learned previously.

- If leading this exercise, the following is to be read out loud:

    1. As you breathe, please visualize, if you will, your breath as white light. Let this breath fill your mind space with white light. (This can be suggested to ASD students as filling a bowl or vase [their minds] with a pure, clean white liquid. Be playful and creative when leading visualizations.)

    2. The white light will fill your mind with brightness and clarity that will expose, reveal, and illuminate any dark shadowy places that may conceal or harbor any negative past thinking such as fearful thoughts, tense feelings, or self-doubt from past experiences. The white light will reveal any thoughts about past victories or defeats, future expectations, or fantasies or thoughts that keep you from being aware of who you are, and what your new options and choices are in the present moment.

    3. As you focus on this visualization, you might find your mind quietening down and becoming more and more grounded. The chattering mind will continue to rattle along, yet this time you are only observing the chatter and not participating with it, or you could imagine that the chattering mind is dissolving and draining out of your life like old, dirty sink water. You can now allow for the departure of any thoughts, voices, and patterns in your mind that in the past kept you from being totally aware of the present moment you were living.

    4. (A teaching mantra) "You control your mind, your mind does not control you. You are in control of your thoughts and focus."

5. Use this visualization wisely and frequently to calm yourself down and to find harmony in yourself, even if it is only for a few precious moments.

6. Slowly, let's come to a close. Please bring your focus to me and slowly open your eyes if your eyes were closed. Thank you.

7. Please finish now with three breaths of *misogi* on your own.

In martial arts or heroic movies, the picture of the serene and confident warrior standing firm before superior numbers, ready to face death with peace in spirit, and clarity and focus in mind, evokes awe and respect. The discipline of "mindfulness" to the present moment allows the hero access to a mental and physiological cohesiveness, allowing them to execute clear, precise, energetic movements to survive the battle.

After years of practice in the martial arts, learning the movements and coping with the physical demands, one may begin to understand the idea that without a calmness of mind and spirit, the martial journey is just as impossible as it seemed on the very first day of practice. This principle applies to any form of learning new information or data.

As a professional dancer and a martial arts practitioner, I am well aware of the pitfalls of mindlessness—"to be without mind". If you forget your steps of the choreography during a performance in front of a large audience, or freeze up mentally in a martial situation, the consequences can be embarrassing and dangerous, not only for yourself but for others as well.

The holistic premise that the mind and body are one implies that what is changed in the mind can affect the body and vice versa. Breath awareness calms and focusses the mind. Therefore, if we focus our minds on the intention to change a particular detrimental behavior, then we are likely to succeed in our endeavors.

I hold this holistic premise to be true and incorporate it into my work with all my clients regardless of whether they are ASD challenged or not. For example, I was working with an ASD adolescent on a challenging movement. When he was frustrated, he would go into fits, start stomping, and become dejected enough to refuse to engage. First, I had the young man remember his breath awareness; this settled him down enough to allow the focus of his breathing to calm and focus his mind. From this cleared space and calmness of mind, we were able to continue the session. He learned that should he become unsettled in his mind while doing anything, he would start from the foundation: (1) Focus on the breath (2) to clear the mind (3) to accomplish what you want.

In working with ASD-challenged young people, I always remind them that, no matter how frustrating their past lives were, the present moment is where all the changes occur. Thus, the practice is to focus on their present moment achievements. The result is their gaining confidence and strength from what they accomplish in the present. Being willing to try their best, and acknowledging their own efforts, is what matters.

As a teacher for 25 years, it does not surprise me that my mentoring and guiding of ASD students and adolescents varies very little from my approach to teaching dancers or students of the martial arts. And the approach is this: when I calm a student's mind down from personal fears and anxieties, I am mostly likely to be successful in helping this student learn and be empowered with what I am teaching.

It is the calming and refocussing of the mind that will lead to the acknowledgment of one's power and intelligence, and the ability to direct this focus to carrying out an intention.

"Clear vase" visualization

This next exercise, the "Clear vase" visualization—a body *misogi*—is an exercise I have found to be very effective in helping individuals begin the process of unifying the breath, mind, and body connection. For instance, in my private practice, I use this visualization in cases in which clients have experienced extreme trauma to their mind or bodies. Cases in which I utilize this exercise have ranged from physical, emotional, and sexual abuse to post-open-heart surgery, from severe knee repair rehabilitation, to a 15-year-old young man with AS who had given up hope that he would ever be coordinated enough to play a team sport or game. Many people with ASD exhibit symptoms of post-traumatic stress disorder. In their case, it is often a result of years of bullying from their peers (Attwood 2006). Repeated trauma results in low self-esteem—a distorted image of a damaged, insufficient, and unlovable sense of self. The "Clear vase" visualization will help the individual to see in their mind's eye a vision of a complete self—not isolated images of pieces and fragments.

When we are injured or sick, we tend to see ourselves in pieces. A broken foot may feel like a separate entity from the rest of our body. The stimulation of pain can alienate the very thing an injured or traumatic person needs: attention to the healing process. I have heard many clients in my private practice speak in a language in which their ailments and challenges were alien beings inside them, yet all along they were talking about their own bodies. This language separates them from a vision of a whole self, and instead creates an experience of fragmentation.

Many ASD individuals unfortunately see themselves in pieces—as uncoordinated, unfocussed, and ungrounded individuals, sometimes desperately trying to make sense of the lives they are living. With some of my older AS clients, 19–23 years old, this dilemma of "not having it together" manifests as a deeper frustration about life, leading to feelings of despair and depression—which in turn show up as lethargic and directionless life-styles of procrastination. The following visualization exercise can begin the process of healing from the toxic language, memories, and visions of their past.

"Clear vase" visualization—the whole mind/body *misogi*

Instructor's notes:

- Begin by doing a series of breath *misogi* exercises as learned previously.

- You could prepare the visualization exercise beforehand by drawing vases and containers on the chalkboard. If leading this exercise, the following is to be read out loud:

  1. Begin, as always, with awareness of how you are breathing. That's right, just breathe in through your nose and gently breathe out of a relaxed mouth and face. Please breathe throughout the following visualization.

  2. You can do this visualization exercise with your eyes closed.

  3. Lie down comfortably (if possible) or rest your head on your desk, or sit comfortably and let's begin.

4. Please visualize, if you will, a clear vase, or something else that holds water or liquid.

5. See the outline, or shape of this vase, in the form of your body. Please take your time to do this.

6. Please see this "body" vase as transparent, as if it was made of clear glass.

7. At the top of this body vase (at the top of your head), there is an opening to pour water or liquid into.

8. Remember to continue to breathe while you are doing this in your mind. Since you can see through your body vase because it is made of glass, you can see your skeletal system, muscles, internal organs, your brain, and so on. You do not need to worry about being anatomically correct. Just see this exercise as simply as you want to see it.

9. Continue to breathe comfortably as you now pick a clear liquid to pour into your body vase.

10. Allow this liquid to be clean and pure. Now, please pick a color that represents optimal health and healing, power and strength. It can be any color you want: gold, green, yellow, blue, whatever color you want.

11. Now, with an endless quantity of this colored liquid, which represents health and healing, power and strength, begin to pour slowly into your body vase from the top.

12. As your body vase begins to fill with this colored liquid you have chosen, it starts to fill from the lowest point first: your feet.

13. Notice that all the inner spaces, crevices, and folds of your body shape are completely submerged in liquid as the level rises. There is no place in your body vase that is left exposed as the colored liquid rises.

14. The liquid level inside your body vase continues to rise, as you slowly and carefully pour your colored liquid in. (Pause in your instruction for everyone to do this part…very important.)

15. You may notice that you may be almost at the top of your body vase.

16. When you finally reach the top of your body vase (the top of your scalp), finish pouring. Should some liquid overflow out of your body vase, that's ok.

17. Now breathe into the vision of your inner body immersed in the healing colored liquid.

18. Notice how your muscles are releasing old stress and gripping as they float in this healing liquid.

19. Notice how your "guts" and your stomach are relaxed and no longer knotted up with anxiety or fear.

20. All your internal body is immersed in this healing and strength-giving liquid.

21. Breathe with this vision of yourself and feel the inner strength inside you.

22. Slowly now, with relaxed breathing, let's finish the visualization.

23. In three rich, deep breaths, gradually open your eyes.

24. Please remember how you feel now and how you felt as you did this visualization.

25. Everyone now please slowly come to standing and finish with three breaths of *misogi*.

———————

4

Standing on Your Own Two Feet

Thus far, I have discussed using breath, *misogi,* and visualization to clear and focus the mind. Without a clear mind, there is no point building up the body. It would be like constructing a house without an architect or an engineer. Once the mind is clear and focussed through breath, we are now in a position to mindfully supervise the construction of an aligned posture. I use this imagery of building a structure with my clients/mentees. I explain to them that without a stable and strong foundation, the structure will collapse over time. In this chapter, I will discuss how to build a strong physical foundation from the ground up.

Hans Asperger noted that the children he observed with characteristics that we now call "Asperger's Syndrome (AS)" were, for the most part, clumsy and uncoordinated. (Asperger 1944). Most of my clients with autistic spectrum disorder (ASD) exhibit signs of one or more of the following: weak muscle development, challenges with motor planning (apraxia), uncoordinated muscle response, poor hand/eye coordination, unsure footing, a sense of imbalance, and poor posture. They often walk with either a sense of lightness, tripping forward on the balls of their feet as if they are floating off the ground, or a heaviness that appears and sounds like they are plodding into the earth. These physiological challenges can be devastating and frustrating to a growing adolescent who can't partici- pate in group social games that may require strength, agility, running, catching, kicking, or other motor skills. I have heard ASD students ratio- nalize their physiological challenges with such statements as, "It doesn't matter: brain over brawn any day" or "Anyway, I don't like physical activi- ties—I find them boring." When I hear this, I know it is sometimes untrue.

I can see in their eyes and read their body language while they watch other kids do what they cannot do—a communication of envy and hopelessness. The ASD individual might confess that they had tried to participate in sports and were chosen last or not chosen at all, laughed at, or bullied off the team. It does not help that many parents fear for their child's safety—because of their clumsiness and weak muscle control. Lacking confidence in their child's ability to overcome their physical challenges, as well as their own ability to teach these skills, some parents give up trying to teach basic activities such as bike riding, ball throwing, ball kicking and catching—basic tools for playing games with other kids and learning to build social relationships from an early age on through adolescence. When I work with ASD teens, I need to coax and assure them to "Please just trust me and I will help you learn what you need to learn so you may feel confident and secure in yourself and your body." I have taught young ASD adults past 17 years old how to ride a bike for the first time.

The adolescent habits of wearing heavy backpacks and sitting in front of computers for hours on end are very damaging positions for their growing bodies (Figures 4.1 and 4.2). I have had numerous cases of male AS clients who must have their backpacks loaded with gaming books, palm pilots and computers wherever they go. For their developing bodies the weight of 20–35 lbs stressing their spines sends their heads so far forward of their torsos that they look like baby vultures even without their backpacks on!

What I have discovered in my years of working with the ASD population is that most of them are disconnected from their bodies. I find this to be very similar to individuals I have worked with who were traumatized by injury, severe or not, or had suffered spiritual, emotional, or physical abuse at any age. Being a survivor of childhood abuse myself, I easily recognize the "floating off the ground," spacey-in-the-head, detached look of "not really being part of this world." When a person is not fully grounded in their body, they may exhibit behaviors that include such things as poor proprioception (difficulty in knowing where one's body is in space when moving around), not following basic personal hygiene concepts, and not being aware of socially acceptable physical displays such as not picking your nose in front of the person you are talking to. The sense of one's own body in relation to others and the world around them is deficient and limited for many of these young folks, leading to social rejection and self-alienation.

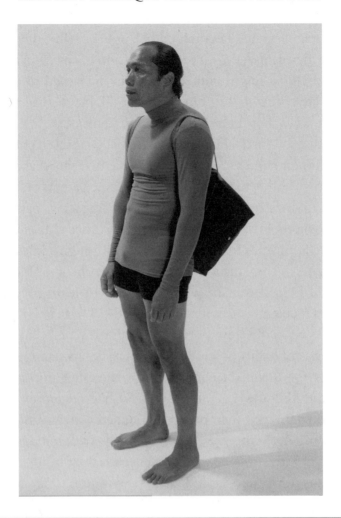

Figure 4.1 Incorrect posture with heavy backpack

I feel that it is crucial for ASD populations in public and private schools to have a physical education program that is both sensitive to and effective for their learning capabilities. Time and time again I have seen in private practice and at school settings that when an individual experiences a sense of being in their body with stability and awareness, the qualities of self-confidence, empowerment, and, most importantly, the display of personal presence in their life is manifested for all to see. All aspects of the individual's life begin to transform and evolve when they have the experience of "I know who I am and I know my power."

Here is a Pathfinder teaching poem:

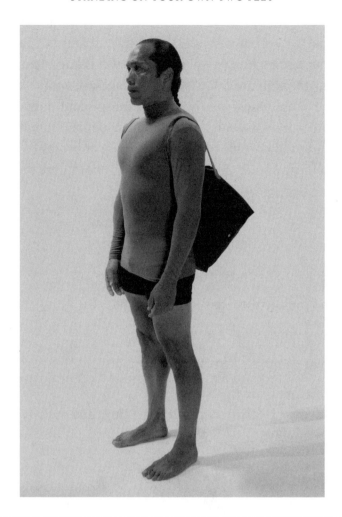

Figure 4.2 Correct posture with heavy backpack

The awareness of your breath keeps you in the present moment.

Breath quiets and focusses the mind.

With a clear disciplined mind you direct your body to do what you want it to do—not what it wants to do without you.

Discipline and focus your mind.

Your mind will lead and heal the body.

"Stand your ground firmly with flexibility." This is a basic Pathfinder training mantra. When we are standing with awareness we are presenting ourselves in our power base—with faith and confidence vibrating through every cell of our bodies. How we present ourselves is important. The impressions we create through our body language make a powerful statement. It is about how we show others how we "stand our ground" literally.

In Pathfinder training one's self-awareness begins from the inside out and from the ground up. One of the first exercise concepts I teach my ASD clients is the "Basic points of alignment." These points are the basic structural plan for building body alignment.

Basic points of alignment

1. Tripod points in the feet (Figure 4.3). They are:

   • point under the large toe metatarsal

   • point under small toe metatarsal

   • point under the heel.

   Visualization:
   Imagine your feet are three-pronged plugs and earth is the outlet.

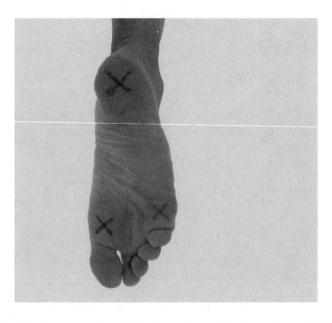

Figure 4.3 Tripod points

Push into these points downwards, as if you are "plugging" into earth.

2. Live feet. Arches activated—this activates the inner thigh muscles, helping in the hip—knee—ankle alignment (Figures 4.4, 4.5).

3. Knees soft and flexible. They are the "shock absorbers" of the body (Figures 4.6, 4.7).

4. The pelvic girdle is allowed to "float" right on top of two legs. This speaks about releasing old tension in the buttocks and lower back (Figures 4.8, 4.9).

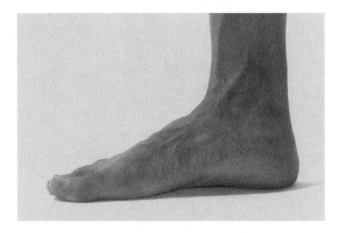

Figure 4.4 "Live feet"—arches activated

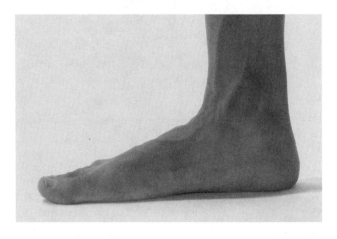

Figure 4.5 "Flat feet"—arches collapsed

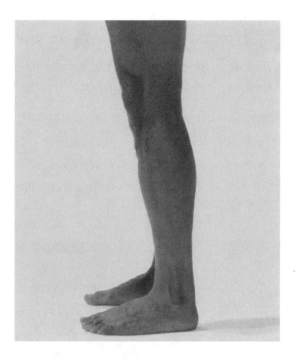

Figure 4.6 "Shock absorber" of knees activated—energy flows through them

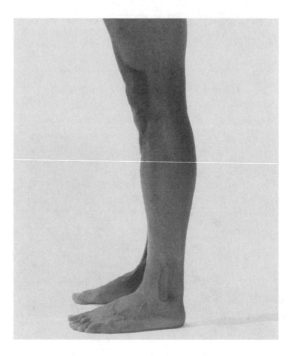

Figure 4.7 Knees locked—energy flow clogged

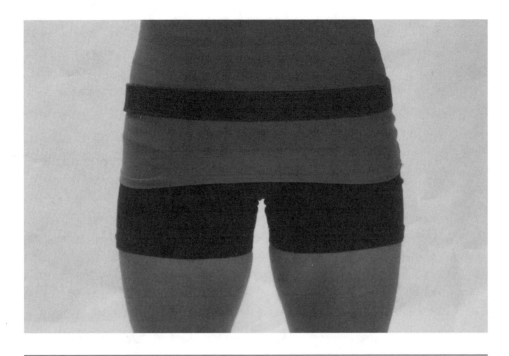

Figure 4.8 Pelvis "floating"—upper body weight in equilibrium on top of two legs

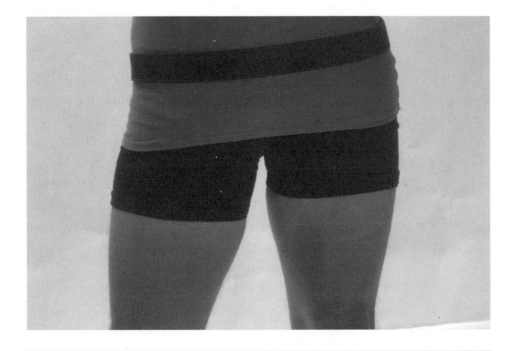

Figure 4.9 Pelvis tilted—weight of upper body lodged into one hip and one leg only

5. Belly breathing into the lower abdominal area. Allow the lungs to inflate and deflate naturally without allowing any gripping or rising of energy to the upper body (i.e shoulders and neck) (Figures 4.10, 4.11). Keep the facial mask relaxed—especially the muscles around the mouth and eyes.

6. The sunburst points. Visualization: Visualize a sunburst—energy expanding outwardly from a central point. There are two points to consider—one sunburst point is located on the breast bone or sternum area and the other sunburst point is located between the shoulder blades. Activate power and the energy of extension from both points equally (Figures 4.12, 4.13). This point is very important in upper body alignment.

7. Relax the neck muscles because now you are aware of dropping energy into the belly.

8. Finally, bring the head back to neutral. "Neutral" is a place where the head sits comfortably right on top of the neck. By using neck and chest muscles properly the head is neither in front of the torso (creating shoulder and lower back pain) or behind the torso (creating sway back, pinching or pain and protruding belly) (Figures 4.14 - 4.20).

Standing with flexibility and alignment in the body will release standing-position fatigue and stress. When you are standing, try to have flexible, unlocked knees. Energetically speaking, with your knees unlocked, your body can draw new energy charge from earth (being grounded) and then, in a circular fashion, drain old, stale energy out through your legs. Imagine releasing the locked knees as "unkinking the hose." When a water hose is kinked the flow of water is diminished or blocked altogether. Unkink the hose and the water flows unhindered. Thus, we improve our posture to allow energy to flow easily through our bodies.

I call this pro-active standing. Pro-active standing shows focus and intention. It demonstrates that you are aware, rather than floating away in daydreams. Your standing posture demonstrates an energetic, dynamic connection to earth. Your standing posture reflects your confidence and power.

Stand tall and breathe!

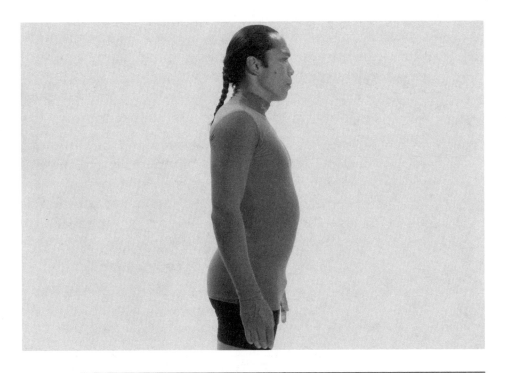

Figure 4.10 Inflate belly on the inhale

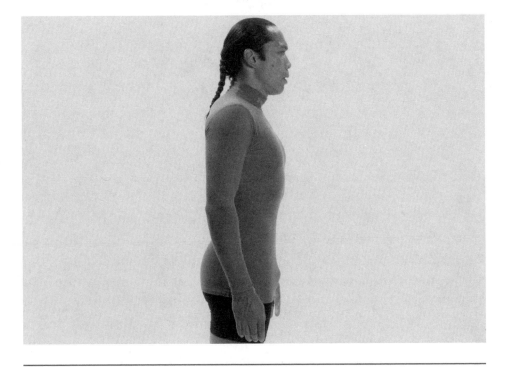

Figure 4.11 Deflate belly on the exhale

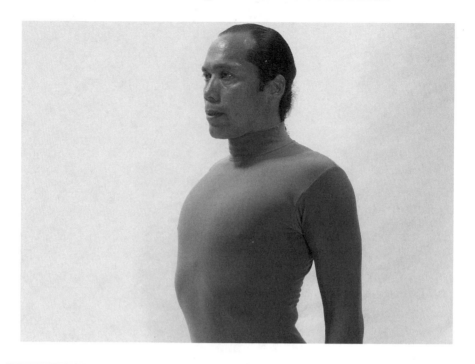

Figure 4.12 Too much energy extended from the sunburst point in the sternum

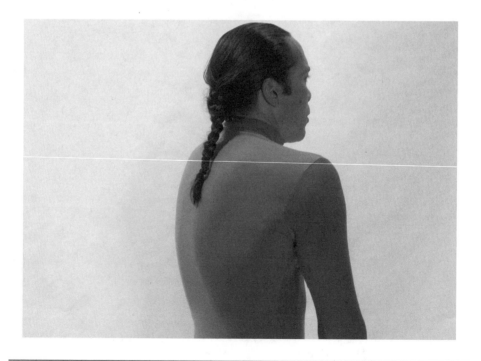

Figure 4.13 Too much energy extended from the sunburst point between the shoulder blades

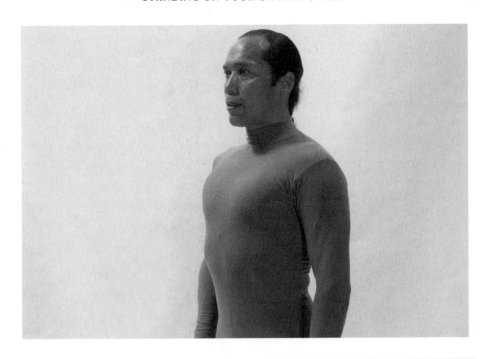

Figure 4.14 Energy extending equally from both sunburst points

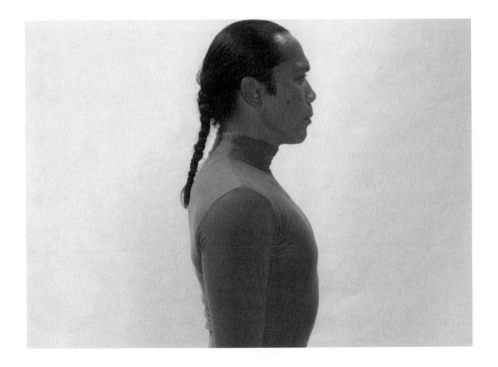

Figure 4.15 Energy extending equally from both sunburst points

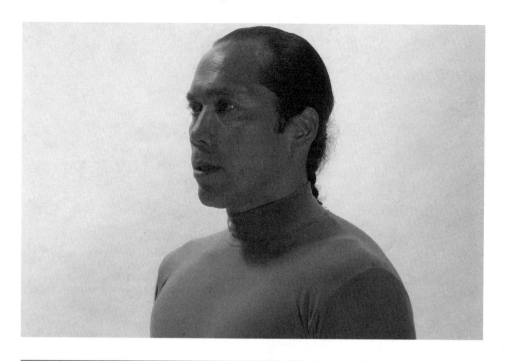

Figure 4.16 Head and neck balanced and aligned

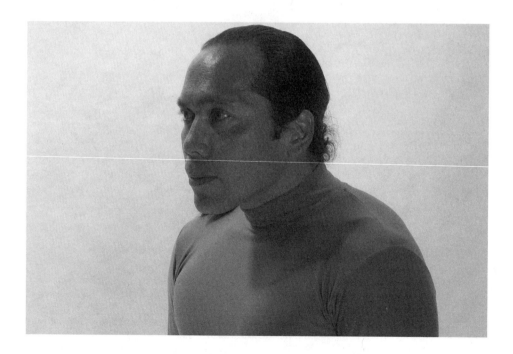

Figure 4.17 Head in front of body—heavy backpacks, watching TV or computers

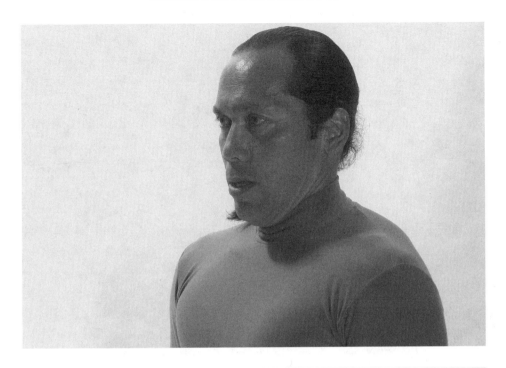

Figure 4.18 Head behind body—knees

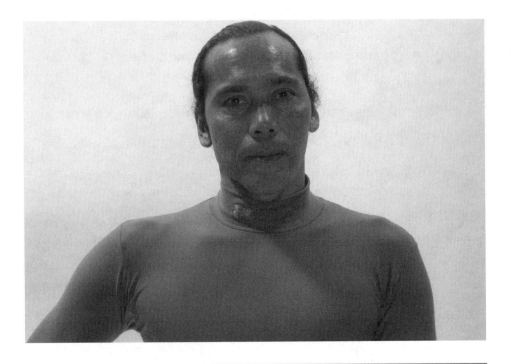

Figure 4.19 Head to one side—usually standing on one leg as well

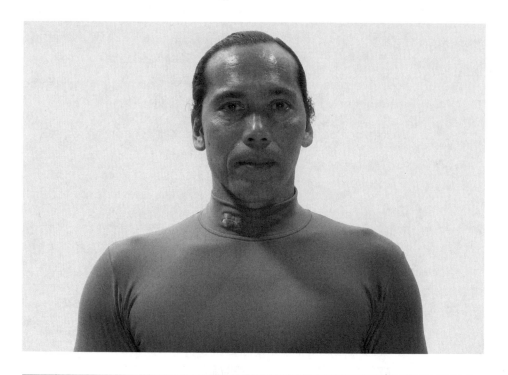

Figure 4.20 Head centred

"Standing your ground" exercise
(posture and the extension of one's energy)

Instructor's notes:

- Begin by doing a series of breath *misogi* exercises as learned previously.

- If leading this exercise, the following is to be read out loud:

  1. Everyone, please do three breaths of *misogi* to clear your mind and settle down in order to learn something new.

  2. Please stand in a powerful warrior stance (Figure 4.21): legs wide apart—comfortable, yet not so wide that you would not lift one foot at a time if you had to.

  3. (Visualization and verbal instruction) You stand in a circle of challenge, surrounded by foes. You are alone and outnumbered. Yet you stand without fear or anxiety. In fact, you express with your whole self the power of confidence and the truth of your inner strength. You draw your energy and power from earth and it travels to the top of your head. You have neither fear nor

doubt in who you are and how capable you are in taking care of the situation at hand.

4. Your eye gaze is straight out in front of you and parallel to the ground. Let your gaze be soft and relaxed.

5. Work your points of alignment (review them for everyone):

   o Tripod points in the feet.

   o Live feet: arches activated—this activates the inner thigh muscles, helping in the knee hip alignment.

   o Soft relaxed ankles.

   o Knees soft and flexible—they are the "shock absorbers" of the body.

   o The pelvic girdle is allowed to "float" right on top of two legs.

   o Belly breathe into your lower abdominal area. Keep the facial mask relaxed: most especially, the muscles around the mouth and eyes.

   o Activate power and energy extension in the sunburst points.

   o Relax the neck muscles.

   o Finally, bring the head back to neutral.

6. Please take a moment to breathe deeply.

7. Now connect to earth through your tripod points in your feet.

8. As you push into the ground, making good connection to earth, breathe deeply as you lengthen your spine and stand tall.

9. Great! Now ignite your sunburst points in your chest and the middle of your back to really open up your posture.

10. You look great! Now remember, as you feel the extension of energy through your chest and back, try to keep your chin down and the back of your neck relaxed.

11. All right, let us hold this posture for three breath cycles.

12. Great. Finish now with three breaths of *misogi*.

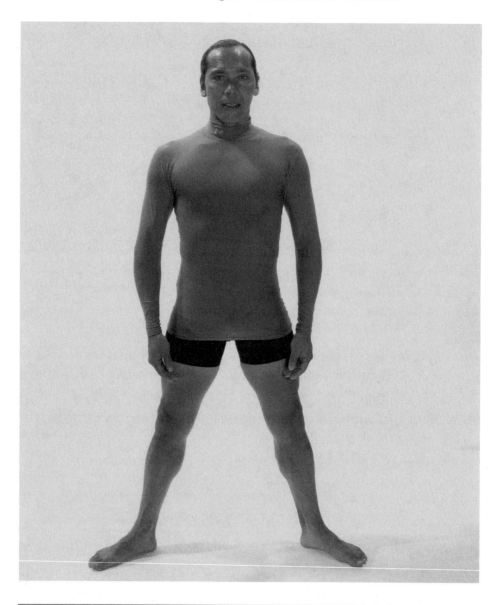

Figure 4.21 Pathfinder warrior stance: legs wide apart—comfortably standing your ground

Instructor's note: This exercise, like most static energy poses, can be used to capture an individual's or a class's attention by requesting "Please stand to ground and focus yourselves before you begin the study session (or test)." When I find a client getting anxious, I will ask them to stand for a quiet moment and do some *misogi* breathing to calm down and know things are safe.

Honoring gravity: Opposition forces at play

This concept speaks about the ability to push downwards (earth bound) to lengthen upwards (heaven bound). The idea of oppositional forces at play within the body is realized by the extension of energy throughout the entire body. It is comparable to how plants grow: establishing a base and foundation by downward-reaching roots with stem and flowers and leaves extending heavenward.

Honoring gravity speaks highly of our connection to earth. Staying grounded through our feet is one way of staying in connection to earth.

The following exercise is an illustration of isometrics: pushing against a stationary object/plane of reference with a complementary force of energy. This concept allows an individual to feel the energetic connection of the body to earth and heaven.

"Making gold coins" exercise

Instructor's notes:

- Begin by doing a series of breath *misogi* exercises as learned previously.

- If leading this exercise, the following is to be read out loud:

  1. Everyone, please do three breaths of *misogi* to clear your mind and settle down so you can learn something new.

  2. Please place your hands together. Position your hands in front of your stomach and then move your hands six inches away from your body, keeping them at the same level (Figure 4.22).

  3. Now visualize, if you will, a tiny ball of gold between your pressed palms.

  4. Now inhale through your nose gently.

  5. Hold it for a second.

  6. And now, as you breathe out of your mouth gently, press your palms together as hard as you can, as if you are making a coin out of that tiny ball of gold (Figure 4.23).

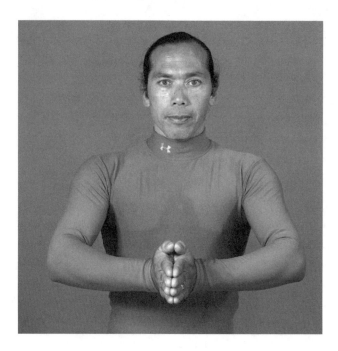

Figure 4.22 Place your hands together—stomach height, hands held away from the body

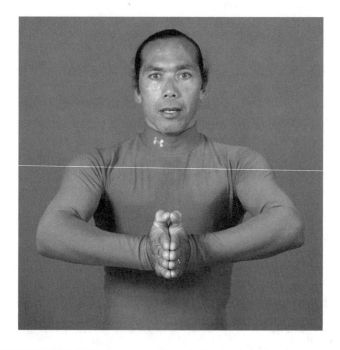

Figure 4.23 Press your palms together strongly, while keeping your shoulders down and your hands held gently away from your body. Keep your focus straight ahead with eyes open

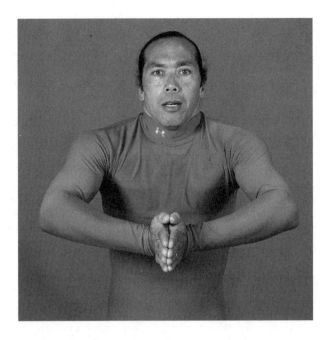

Figure 4.24 Incorrect: Stressing neck and shoulders by allowing the shoulders to rise towards the ears and the chin jutting upwards while pressing palms together

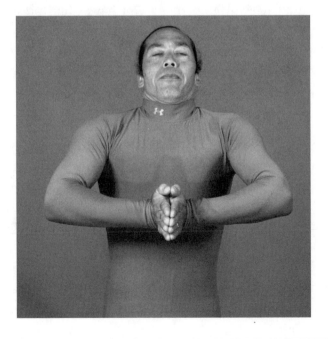

Figure 4.25 Incorrect: Trying too hard with shoulders raised and with eyes closed—losing connection to what is going on

7. Good! Let's try it again. This time, let's think of keeping our shoulders down when we press our palms together. Let's use our upper back and chest to feel the power of our pressing. Ok. Let's go!

8. Everyone making gold coins! Are you feeling the energy in your upper back and chest? Keep those shoulders down while you are pressing your palms together (Figures 4.24, 4.25). Great!

9. Easy does it with your head when you are pressing your palms together. Try to keep your head right where it is and not in front of your torso or behind. Use only your chest and upper back to do the pressing.

10. Let's finish now with three breaths of *misogi*.

———————

Instructor's note: Now try the "Standing your ground" exercise again. This time the points we want to feel "pressing" are the tripod points of the feet into earth. Like plugging into earth. The feet are the three-prong plugs and earth is the outlet. Get grounded! As you have them press their tripod points of their feet into the ground, use the pushing down energy to lengthen their backs and necks upwards at the same time. Oppositional forces at play. Have them try and "touch" the tops of their heads to the sky! This will initiate a nice long spine and proper posture without stress in their bodies.

Special training note for parents, teachers and mentors: The wisdom from being grounded

In the creation of any relationship there is connection. A meeting must occur at some level in order to create a place of interaction, which then allows for a deeper connection.

In the verbal communication between two people, tools for connecting include the action of speaking and perhaps more important, active receptive listening.

As Pathfinders, teachers, parents, and caregivers, we listen for clues in the individual's journey to see how best to lead them. We see how best we can find a path for their development.

Listening takes great patience and awareness on our part. We must be grounded in our emotional and physical energies in order to be able to listen to someone else's needs, anxieties, and fears besides our own. Mentoring an anxious and worried AS teen to listen and be more aware of another's feelings, especially if there is conflict, is to ask the AS teen to be grounded, prepared to listen and able to respond from a level-headed place. I do not know many "neuro-typicals" who can do this!

Breathing and staying charged in the body helps tremendously. Being grounded in our physical and emotional bodies allows us to drop our preconceived ideas and be open to dialogue. It is from this wisdom of staying grounded that we can truly hear the individual's pain, anxiety, stress, and frustrations. Then we are able to validate their experience, which is the first step in making a connection with another person. Once we have joined with another in their experience, we gain their trust. When we have trust we now may begin to offer help and mentorship.

I listen and learn.

When mentoring or teaching, I listen and provide the "witness" so that the mentee/student can express openly and freely. I release the need to rush in and fix everything when I listen to their complaints and fears from a grounded supportive place.

Thus, as Pathfinders, mentors, healers, or teachers, we allow for the individual to feel the "heat" of their own evolving thinking process, as well as their emotional and behavioral growing pains. We give them honored space so that they can learn and grow.

When speaking, always speak with breath, space, and a sense of timing. Timing is knowing when to say what needs to be said with the power and insight to help the student learn and grow. Slow down your presentation! This applies most importantly when emotions are high and you are the one who is supposed to be in the driver's seat. Take your emotions out of the heat of the moment and listen carefully to their confusion, fear, anxiety, or anger. Stay grounded in your own breathing and how you communicate through your body language.

It is important to have a solid connection to earth under your feet, whether you are standing or sitting, as you speak. Sit on your throne or stand your ground.

To conclude, staying grounded is as important, if not more so, for the teachers, parents, and mentors, as it is for our students/mentees.

Do not waste the opportunity to forge the bonds of connection *in the moment*.

5

Posture, Presence, and Extension

Posture, presence, and extension are three very important physical and energetic components in my work with all my clients. Posture, presence, and extension are the non-verbal forms through which our inner selves—personality, emotions, moods, character, and energy—are expressed. Whether we are aware of it or not, how we stand, sit, and move energy though our bodies has an immediate and direct effect on ourselves and on those around us.

When we interact with others we exchange energetic charge—giving and receiving energy (*ki, chi*). We affect each other by the moods we are in, and especially how we present ourselves and offer ourselves to others during interactions, no matter how brief. For example, when a clerk in a store gives us a warm welcome, our spirits are lifted, and we are more likely to give a warm welcome to the next person we meet. Energy gets transmitted from one person to the next, similar to a chain reaction.

Understanding and practicing posture, presence, and extension is vital in order to express oneself to the highest potential and to interact with others beneficently.

Posture

Posture is the outcome of skeletal muscle responses to a command from the brain to find harmony with gravity and physical equilibrium with one's physical environment. Posture is also affected by one's inner state and past history.

O'Sensei, said in his poem teachings, "A good stance and posture reflect a proper state of mind" (Stevens 1992). I find these words to ring true.

The downward pulling of gravity on the body can result in a collapse in posture if one is not vigilant in mind/body to prevent it. This collapse in posture will eventually block the energy pathways that course through the entire body. This phenomenon can be compared to the kinking of a water hose by bending it and decreasing the flow of water. When explaining posture and flow of energy to my students with autistic spectrum disorder (ASD), I draw on the board a straight garden hose and then a second garden hose that is all twisted up and kinked. The illustration is plain to see: water (energy) flows through the unkinked hose, moving with power, harmony, and ease. The twisted and kinked hose jams the water (energy) flow to a trickle or non-flow. Energy can be illustrated as electrical, wind, or water. Any illustration that presents flow and stagnation will do.

Common areas for stagnant energy in the body due to poor posture, or "kinking of the hose" are the lower back or hip joints—which in turn will aggravate the shoulders and neck alignment, stressing muscle and tiring the whole system. When the flow of your life force (energy) is compromised, movement of vital information and stimulation needed to function in daily living is also compromised—even the smallest amount of blockage could be enough to have an effect. In time, these blockages can grow into something more serious that threatens one's health and well-being.

Emotional health, past history, and self-concept affect one's posture, presence, and extension. Thus, any trauma that a young person with Asperger's Syndrome (AS) may have experienced at a young age is likely to have become anchored in their body and will show up in how they carry themselves and express themselves physically. For example, they might be hunched over in the shoulders, ready to protect themselves from abuse, or to try to appear invisible, withdrawing from unwanted attention by others, such as teasing or bullying.

Posture is also affected by daily activities. For example, relationship to gravity is challenged by the heavy backpacks adolescents carry to school these days. Self-esteem, feeling uncomfortable about their growing bodies during puberty, trying to mimic the social physical mannerisms of their "cool friends," and weight issues also affect posture. Even fashion, such as the recently popular baggy pants look, can be disruptive for hip alignment, walking stride, and vertical alignment. These issues are often compounded in those with ASD who already have tendencies towards poor body awareness, weak musculature, quirky running and walking gaits, and a collapse in the chest and torso region.

The collapse in body posture inhibits energy flow throughout the whole mind/body affording even less juice for the emotional and cognitive well-being of the AS student, especially when that student is under stress and anxious. I found in my work with AS males ages 14 yearsand older that if they are in poor physical health they are more likely to have symptoms of depression. The mind/body connection, a well-documented phenomenon in health research, is a salient issue for most if not all individuals with AS. Breathing into a body with good posture is the first step towards improving one's health, life, and social relationships.

Basic floor exercise (for the upper back)

This exercise is one in a series of exercises that is done lying on the ground. From this prone position, clearing body alignment from the effects of twisting, collapsing, or caving in can be discovered without the stress of the downward force of gravity. This particular exercise will focus on the shoulders and head, although the whole body is considered as well.

Instructor's notes:

- Lying on the floor is a must. This would be a good exercise to do on a rug or yoga mat in an open space or gym.

- Equipment needed is a three-ft dowel purchased from a lumberyard or hardware store. If none is available, a belt or a towel held taut between the hands will suffice.

- If leading this exercise, the following is to be read out loud:

    1. Please, everyone, do three breaths of *misogi* to clear your mind and settle down so you can learn something new.

    2. Please lie down on your back and hold the dowel across your thighs.

    3. Bring your knees in close to your body with your feet engaging the floor.

    4. While lying on your back begin to activate your "belly breath."

5. That's right. Fill your belly—on the inhale—like a balloon. Then gently let your belly flatten on your exhale.

6. Great. Please continue breathing this way as you do this exercise now.

7. I would like you now to see how heavy you can make your shoulder blades… just let them "sink" into the ground (Figure 5.1). Nice. This connection to the ground with your shoulder blades allows you now to open your chest.

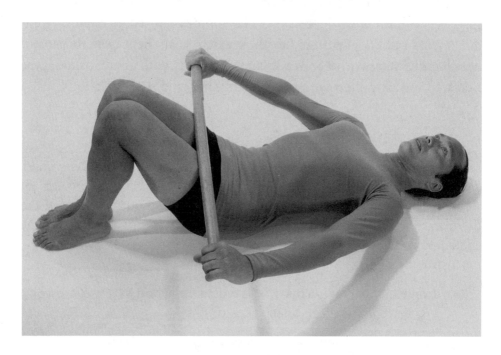

Figure 5.1 Lying with heavy shoulder blades—belly breathing—and mindful focus

8. Great! Continue to relax and "sink" your shoulders to the ground throughout the entire exercise. Keep the connection.

9. Please extend your arms as you hold the dowel firmly.

10. Now, as you *inhale* through your nose—pause and check your shoulder connection to the ground. Now, as you *exhale*—please slowly raise the dowel up and over your head until it touches the floor above your head (Figures 5.2, 5.3), while keeping your

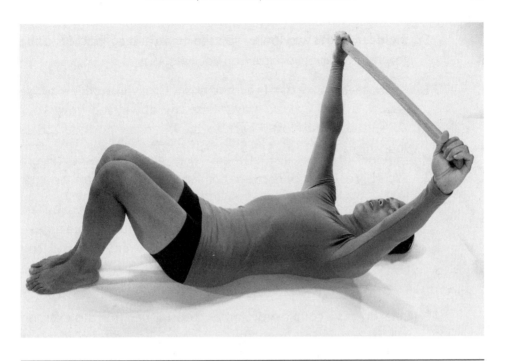

Figure 5.2 Lifting the dowel on the exhale…

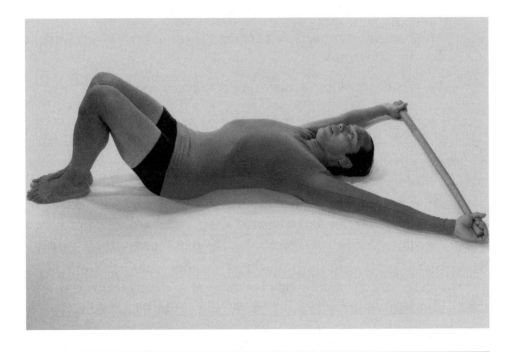

Figure 5.3 …until arms are overhead and backs of the hands are touching the floor

shoulder blades and lower rib cage down and connected to the ground.

11. *Inhale* gently now through your nose, filling your belly—pause —now, as you *exhale*, slowly raise the dowel and bring your arms, hands, and dowel back to the beginning position across your thighs (Figures 5.4, 5.5).

12. Wow! That is a lot of things to do. Yet, everyone did well trying.

13. The main points to this exercise are: (1) Move only on the exhale (2) Keep your shoulders relaxed into the floor the whole time— especially when you are moving your arms over your head, and (3) Breathe! With breathing you reap the benefits of the exercise.

14. Let's do this a couple more times. You will find that this exercise will really help you open up your upper back and shoulders, as well as your chest and arms.

15. Please let's do this again (repeat three–five times).

16. Ok, everyone, let's find a closing to this exercise.

17. Please do three breaths of *misogi* to finish as you lie there without arm movement.

18. Thank you. I hope you feel better now in your body.

———————

Remember this one basic floor exercise. There are many ways to utilize the floor to release stress and load on the body. Enjoy.

When we are in a posture of alignment and aware of ourselves spatially, we allow the body to reclaim a flow of energy, which will re-establish a healthy environment of equilibrium for the mind/body to function in. Renewed energy flow affects the quality of balance in the student. What is done to one part of the mind/body will inevitably affect the other parts of the mind/body. We are whole beings. We are not bits and pieces. This is what is meant by holistic health.

The posture one takes is symbolic of one's self-confidence and awareness or the lack thereof. My dance teacher once said to me, "Ron,

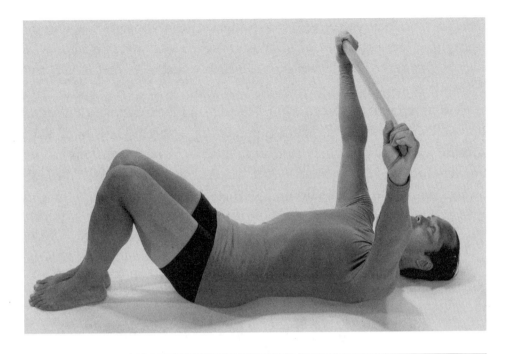

Figure 5.4 On the exhale breath, lift arms off floor...

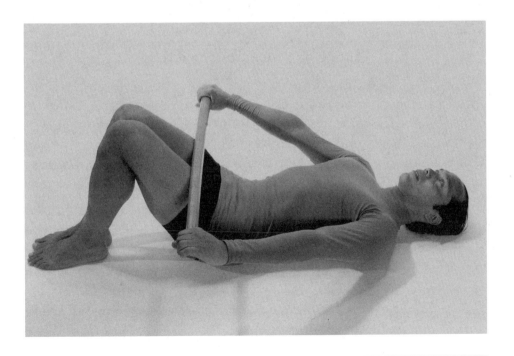

Figure 5.5 ...until arms are back to neutral with dowel across thighs

once you are a dancer, you are always a dancer." Since that time, almost 27 years ago, I am conscious of my posture when walking into a room of people. *First impressions are important.* This is a valuable lesson for ASD and AS adolescents. Our postures show others who we are.

Ask yourself: Do I slouch while I stand? Do I lock my knees and stand upon one leg so that my back is rigid and tight and my hips hurt? Do I breathe up into my shoulders or into my belly? These questions can be answered and the detrimental body behaviors can be transformed through awareness and discipline in training. There is power and significance in these sayings:

- "Stand on your own two feet!"

- "Get a backbone!"

Or in the heat of battle:

- "Stand your ground!"

These words inspire us to express behaviors of courage and bravery, as we are called forth to awaken and be vibrantly alive.

"Sitting on your throne" exercise

The next exercise focusses on what I call pro-active sitting. This exercise will introduce proper muscle awareness while sitting to release fatigue and aching in the neck and shoulders. Using a simple visualization to illustrate empower-ment while sitting, students will look at their alignment in a brand new light. This exercise can be used in a classroom to stimulate awareness for an upcoming challenging lesson, for instance, or to recharge the students if they have been sitting and working hard for a long time.

Instructor's notes:

- Have chairs available to sit on.

- If leading this exercise, the following is to be read out loud:

  1. Begin with breath *misogi* to clear and prepare yourself to try something new.

  2. Please sit down and follow my instructions.

3. I want you to try something new in how you sit. Please adjust your position so that you sit more towards the front edge of the chair, not relying on the chair backrest for support (Figure 5.6).

4. Now separate your legs so that they are hip-width apart, feet uncrossed and planted into the ground. Tripod points of the feet engaging earth.

5. Great. Please place your hands on your thighs gently—palms facing down.

6. (Verbal visualization and instruction) Please visualize this, if you will: You are a fair and generous ruler (King or Queen). You are strong in spirit, mind, and body. You are sitting on your throne with pride, energy, and honor in front of your people—your kingdom. Sit as if you are showing your kingdom how proud you are of them (Figures 5.7, 5.8, 5.9. 5.10). Breathe into your sitting posture gently and powerfully.

7. Great. All of you look like proud and fair Kings (and Queens).

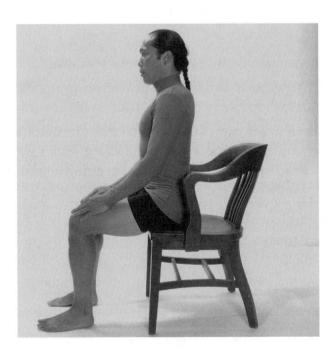

Figure 5.6 Not relying on the back rest to test posture

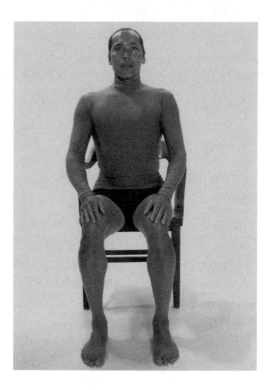

Figure 5.7 *"Sitting on your throne" position*

8. Remember to maintain solid contact with the floor through your feet so you may ground your energy. Let your breathing help you with your posture.

9. Some of you might feel tired after doing this. Don't worry about a thing. It is because you are building your back muscles and stomach muscles. This will help you change your sitting posture. It takes time to get stronger.

10. Great work and concentration! This is not easy to do. You guys did great in trying this out. Thank you. From now on, when I remind you to sit on your throne, you will know what I am talking about. Thank you again.

11. Finish by slowly coming to standing.

12. Please do three breaths of *misogi* to anchor the information into your body.

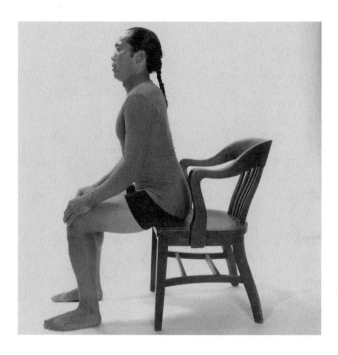

Figure 5.8 Incorrect sitting posture: Head and upper body in front of center line

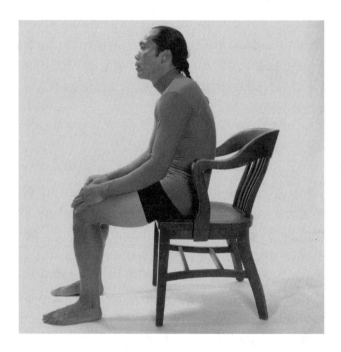

Figure 5.9 Incorrect sitting posture: Collapsed stomach muscles—lower back, neck stressed

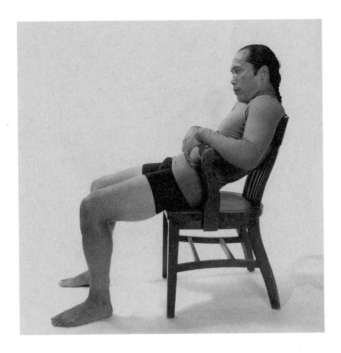

Figure 5.10 Incorrect sitting posture: The "whatever" slouch

Instructor's note: You can use this exercise to gain your students' attention if they have been sitting too long, or to gain their attention at a crucial part of a lesson: "Please sit on your throne before the test so you may settle and be grounded and relaxed." It is also a good position for working at the computer.

Presence

Presence is a quality of being that any dancer or performer knows well. Athletes, martial artists, military leaders, teachers, speakers, and those who lecture in front of large crowds are familiar with the power of one's presence. Presence displays one's confidence, power, and grace. People read presence in others. People identify with those who display a presence that is safe, genuine, and truthful—a presence that lacks pretense—and therefore they themselves feel safe to trust. Like all mammals, we go through the dance of establishing alpha/delta relationships through body language, posture, and how we project our presence.

The concept of presence is very important to introduce to ASD individuals in order for them to become empowered. When people are able to display presence outwardly, they experience an energetic charge generating greater strength to change detrimental behaviors or to face life transitions.

Unfortunately, many ASD people have lived a life of disappointments, bullying, loneliness, and even misunderstanding from those close to them. As a result, they can barely lift their heads away from their computers, video games, daydreams, or other distractions in a vain attempt to fill the void in their own presence. Some AS clients I have worked with had such withdrawn presences that they seemed like wisps of mist entering a room—no one noticed them. You recognize them in the corners of a room of people—how they stand apart from others, involved with themselves or the floor that they stare at. These individuals project very little energetic charge for anyone to pick up on, and therefore there is no viable interface created to establish opening communication, which leads to beginning a relationship.

In developing the awareness of presence for an AS mentee, I start by grounding and charging the inner strengths that are most basic to them. For instance, "You are a good thinker and strategist to play those challenging computer games for hours. You also have a good heart and you show it by your concern for your parents. You are brave to challenge some of your behaviors that you know held you back in the past." And so on. As I strengthen their basic core awareness of themselves, I also begin at the same time to awaken their awareness of their body. Coordinating the development of physical balance, strength, coordination, and grace with core ego (self) building has produced amazing results in the evolution of the AS mentee.

Presence is a dynamic connection of inner strength—the confidence and faith in oneself to be brave and to persevere—with those of the outer energetic and physical expressions. The fruits of such a combination are the strength and integrity to evolve and mature to a place of independence, self-reliance, and the ability to show oneself to others, opening the doors to social connection.

Character mimic exercise

This is a theater exercise I used for years to warm a class up before a rehearsal and now apply to teach presence to my AS mentees. The exercise teaches how different character types are expressed through the human body. This can be a very fun and explorative game to release tension and loosen up.

Instructor's note: If leading this exercise, the following is to be read out loud:

1. Before we begin, please clear the slate in your mind/body by doing three breaths of *misogi* exercises to prepare yourself.

2. This exercise is going to demonstrate different ways in which we project energy in our bodies.

3. Everyone please stand and make a loose line. We are going to play a character I choose and see how we can express that character in our bodies. Everyone imagine a "super hero" character you know and show me how the character looks with all the physical mannerisms, postures, and ways of moving that you can remember.

4. (They will show) Great! Does anyone want to pick another character we can try to mimic? If no one suggests anything, "Ok, how about we all try 'Darth Vader'!"

5. Ready, go! Be the Darth Vader character with all that you can remember about him.

6. Great! Now I want you to show your personal character. Either show who you are or who you want to be someday. Take a moment to visualize this vision of yourself. Ready. Ok, show your character.

7. Do as many characters as you want. Here are some suggestions for characters: the President, a famous rock and roll star, an old man, a shy kid, a *samurai*, and so on. The more outlandish the character the better!

8. Ok, everyone, let's find a closing to this exercise by doing three breaths of *misogi*.

9. Thank you.

———————

Extension

Extension to a dancer means to express a movement, posture, or gesture to the highest and fullest energetic quality possible. I once opened a dance performance with my back to the audience for the first ten minutes of the choreography. I was told in learning the dance piece to "Extend your energy out of your back as if you were facing the audience." To me as a dancer, extension meant to perform at a high level of expression.

In the martial arts, extension refers to the ability to reach beyond the physical limitations without losing one's center of balance. For instance, in weapon training with the *bokken* (wooden swords), a sense of extension will help for fuller cuts with less fatigue and usage of strength. Extension allows for the mind/body to function and flow past points of resistance with safety and effectiveness.

Extension can also be used to describe being more of yourself. I have had many cases of 19–23-year-old AS male clients wanting to learn how to be more of who they are and not to be held back by old patterns. They ask specifically to know how to be more powerful and confident in learning the social "dance" one has to perform in almost all levels of society. From the workplace and the college classroom to casual friendships and budding intimate relationships, extension is a concept that is indispensable to anyone trying to catch up socially with their peers.

Extension also means coming out of our shells and actually take chances. An individual extends themselves in order to start up a dialogue with someone of interest. For someone with AS, this is especially challenging because it does not come naturally or easily. For such folks, coming out of their built-up comfort zones of safety and seclusion is an incredible act of bravery and a milestone in their lives. Extension also means expressing one's spirit and intention through physical bearing and effective dynamic movement.

Extension helps understand how to express personal presence through movements such as balancing, running, jumping, leaping, or just simply standing in a calm fearless manner.

"Unbreakable arm" exercise

This is an excellent demonstration of the power of extension. I learned this from the martial art of *aikido*. It is very simple and yet it speaks volumes about the power of extension and mindfulness.

Instructor's note: If leading this exercise, the following is to be read out loud:

1. Before we begin, please clear the slate in your mind/body by doing three breaths of *misogi* exercises to prepare.

2. Ok. This exercise demonstrates the concept of extension through our bodies.

3. Volunteer? (Choose a student.) Great. Please come up and stand in front of the class.

4. Now, please stand comfortably and hold out one arm.

5. Good. Now, as I try to push down your arm, resist without trying too hard or fighting me. (Push gently down on the student's outstretched arm. The arm will slowly descend due to your downward pressure. If the student resists you by raising their shoulder to brace or holding their breath to maintain the arm strength, that is not the point. The arm will go. Try a couple of times.) (Figures 5.11 and 5.12)

6. Now, try this. Extend your arm and open your fingers of your hand. Breathe in gently. Now, as you breathe out gently, imagine beams of light shooting out of your fingertips (Figure 5.13). Ready?

7. Now, I will try to push your arm down again and let's see what will happen. (What will happen is that as you apply gentle downward pressure on their extended arm, while they are extending their mind and energy through their arm, you will not be able to push their arm down. Try it a couple of times. Remember gentle force from you and relaxed extension from the student.)

8. Anyone else?

9. (After you are done.) Everyone, please do three breaths of *misogi* to anchor this information into your body.

10. Thank you. That was the "Unbreakable arm" exercise.

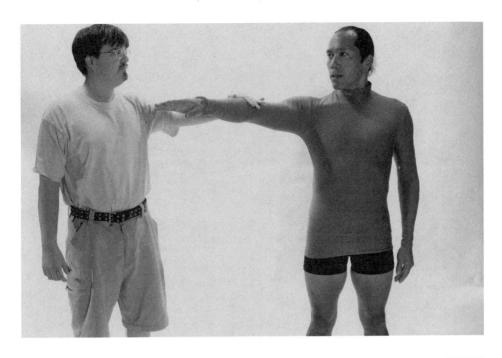

Figure 5.11 Hold the arm out comfortably…and resist the gentle downward pressure

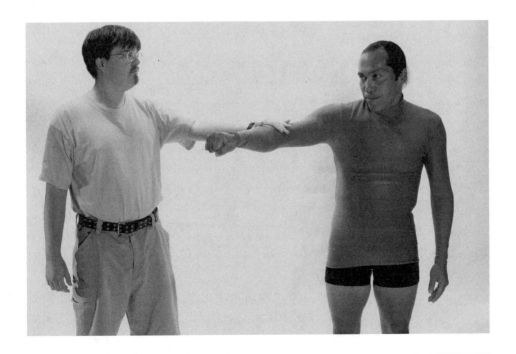

Figure 5.12 Incorrect resisting of downward force

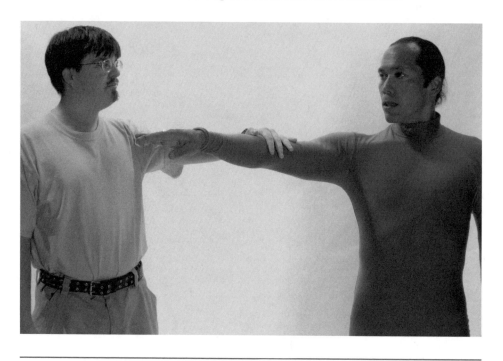

Figure 5.13 Beams of light out of fingertips—relaxed breath out—easily extend through the downward pressure

Art of balancing

To some people, balancing is a circus act: it seems so out of reach that to even suggest it seems comical. Others take to balancing like a fish to water. Balancing and being centered are inherent capabilities in all of us. It is a matter of training to rediscover that essence of being "one" literally.

For persons with ASD, and AS, the act of balancing is a very important step towards centering their minds as well as their bodies. For an adolescent with ASD, being able to control one's balance opens doors to social events such as playing catch, running around, soccer, hiking, hitting an object (tennis ball, volley ball etc.), and dancing. Most importantly, having sound balance allows one to feel confident and relaxed during any movement.

The act of balancing really does ask us to see and embrace being "one" to develop and strengthen a holistic image and awareness of the self as one complete entity. Being "one" means that a person breathes and moves as one piece, thinks as one piece and sees themselves as whole, rather than in pieces. Balancing is a sign of internal discipline and cohesiveness—to be clear in the mind and releasing fear-inducing thoughts of "I can't do it."

Dancers train to balance. As with athletes, gymnasts, trapeze artists, acrobats, and martial artists, every gesture of a dancer is a study of lining up and utilizing the power of being "one." Utilizing this concept, a dancer appears graceful and in full command of their physical power and abilities in a performance. A dancer's training is hard and demanding for this reason.

I find in my work with youngsters, teens, and adults that, when the act of balancing has been achieved, the entire demeanor of the person changes from one of uncertainty of the self and an expectation of failure to a joyful, personal victory of achieving the impossible. Balancing evokes personal pride. To balance is to know the potential of one's power and confidence and be able to show it. Again, balancing is to feel and express neither fear nor self-doubt.

As a rookie dancer in training at the Alvin Ailey School of American Dance in New York City in the late 1970s, I was constantly reminded by my dance teachers to not try so hard when learning to turn or to pirouette. I would learn that it was not a question of physical strength in doing a double or triple or any multiple pirouettes: it was, rather, finding a point of reference—the wooden floor or the stage—and from using that point of reference to stay connected to and use the power of being grounded. Once the opening movement of a turn was created, breaking inertia and initiating turning on a demi-pointed foot, the remaining process required staying aware of not allowing my body parts (arms and head) to flay around causing disruption in my balance, but rather to stay connected to my center (my spine), as well as maintaining posture (a shape or form or pose) in my body. The window of time to complete a single pirouette is less than a second!

Learning how to do a pirouette, I tried and cried and crashed, bashed and bruised my way while my teachers watched and offered their help. After taking pity on me, the ballet master offered this advice:

Relax, you are trying too hard, you have enough strength in your turns for a quadruple pirouette—go back and study the single pirouette. You also keep falling because you are losing contact with the floor. Maintain balance as you spot your head turn. Ron, you must clean up your spotting with more intention.

In time, I managed triple and quadruple pirouettes without making a silly basket case out of myself. Lesson learned. I survived another day of dance training.

Basic balancing exercise

Instructor's notes:

- Have sturdy chairs available to use as balancing aides.

- If leading this exercise, the following is to be read out loud:

    1. Begin with three breaths of *misogi* to clear the slate and prepare yourself for anything.

    2. This exercise will teach you about balancing. I know some of you are already getting anxious and nervous about this. Please know you do not need to be perfect; this is not about being better than someone else or competing with someone else.

    3. It is completely all right if you fall off balance. Stay relaxed and try it again—that is what practicing something is all about.

    4. Ok, let's begin. Everyone stand next to a chair.

    5. Some will think this too easy but please follow my directions anyway. Thank you.

    6. First, stand firmly on two legs. (Note: review the points of alignment.)

    7. Now place one hand on the chair (Figure 5.14).

    8. Gaze at a point directly in front of you, parallel to the ground. Be aware of letting your gaze fall towards the ground, for if you look down you will go down!

    9. The leg closest to the chair will be known as your "standing leg."

    10. The leg farther from the chair will be known as your "working leg."

    11. Slowly shift your body weight to your standing leg.

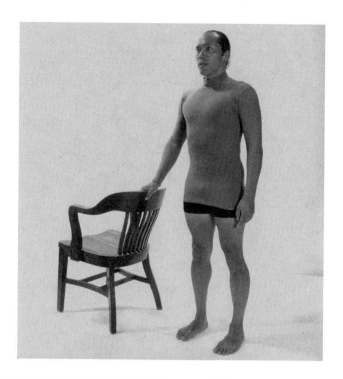

Figure 5.14 Using a chair as a tool to build confidence...why stress?

12. Now, slowly push into the ground through the foot of your standing leg in order to stay tall in your body. (Note: review the "Making gold coins" exercise: To balance: push downward into earth as you lengthen your spine [posture] toward heaven.)

13. Now, calmly lift your outside foot (the working leg side) to a position you can hold comfortably (Figure 5.15).

14. Balance for one breath count.

15. Good! Slowly lower the foot back on the ground.

16. (Check in with the class.) Ok, I saw some of you did fine and others had some challenges. Here are some reminders:

17. Stay connected to the ground by using "making gold coins" energy in your standing leg and foot.

18. Try to use your body as one piece when balancing. Maintain strength in your posture so you do not allow your body alignment to throw you off balance.

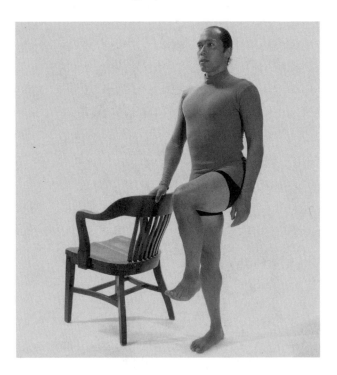

Figure 5.15 Now calmly lift your outside foot (the working leg side) to a position you can hold comfortably

19. And remember: breathe while you are doing this exercise. This keeps your body flexible to make adjustments needed when balancing. Holding your breath makes your body rigid and tight: a good recipe for losing balance.

20. Let's all try this again; then we will switch sides and try the other leg.

21. Ok. Switch legs by standing on the other side of the chair.

22. Great! Remember now: your standing leg is the leg closest to the chair and the working leg is the leg farther from the chair.

23. Here we go: slowly shift your body weight to your standing leg.

24. Now, slowly push into the ground through the foot of your standing leg in order to stay tall in your body (Note: review "Making gold coins" exercise).

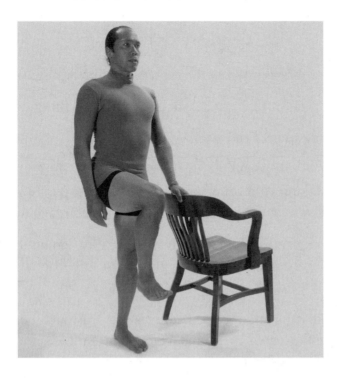

Figure 5.16 Working the other leg—always to both sides of the body

25. Now, calmly lift your outside foot (the working leg side) to a position you can hold comfortably (Figure 5.16).

26. Balance for one breath count.

27. Great! You guys are getting better. Let's try it again.

28. Ok. Everyone, let's find a closing to this exercise by doing three breaths of *misogi*.

29. Thank you everyone for trying and being cool about it.

———————

(As the students get better, increase the time holding the balance to two, then three breath cycles and so on. Challenge them with sensitivity. For those having trouble with this exercise, keep them relaxed and out of their self-critical heads by doing *misogi*.)

Checklist for balancing

1. Relaxed breathing into the center: belly breathing.

2. Mind clear of fear and self-doubt: *misogi* breathing techniques.

3. Body awareness and stability:

   ○ Keep grounded to earth: oppositional forces at play—the "Making gold coins" exercise. To balance: push downward into earth as you lengthen your spine (posture) toward heaven.

   ○ Energize the whole body for stability: points of alignment awareness, especially plugging those tripod points of the feet into earth.

4. Remain calm and focussed. You can get frustrated but don't allow yourself to have a "meltdown." Stay calm: getting anxious will make you lose your balance for sure.

5. Gaze at a point directly in front of you, parallel to the ground. Be aware of not letting your gaze fall towards the ground, for if you look down—you will go down!

What my dance teacher said boiled down to these notes on balancing that I have used ever since:

1. Relax—don't try so hard—trust yourself.

2. Remember the basics—release your ego from doing too much.

3. Be earth friendly and maintain contact to earth—stay grounded.

4. Have a firm intention and resolve to succeed— release fear.

I remind my clients constantly that balancing is a powerful example of synchronizing mind and body with breath and the power of fearlessness. Our emotional integrity, how we feel about ourselves and perceive ourselves, is in cohesion with our body's actions. Thus, to balance is to consolidate all aspects of the whole self. Though we experience balancing as a bodily phenomenon, always remember that your body is just part of the expression of balancing. Balancing incorporates breath/spirit, a focussed mind, clear physical alignment, isometric pushing, and extension of will and energy. All the previous lessons thus far are integrated in order to direct and command your body to balance. Balancing takes entire self-awareness to achieve. Lesson learned.

Also, I find it important to remind my students and clients about the process of learning something new. Learning new information can be hard or easy, so in order to keep at bay the self-critical voice in our minds, remember:

- Lighten up!

- Be compassionate and patient with yourself when learning something new.

- We are supposed to make mistakes while trying. that is why it is called "practice."

- That is why in the beginning it is "learning it" instead of "knowing it."

- Make mistakes and then adjust until you get it.

- Be kind to yourself.

To conclude, learning posture, presence, and extension brings the ASD individual to a new level of self-awareness and empowerment. When applied in daily movement and in the actions of mind/body, posture, presence, and extension define how we express ourselves physically and, more significantly, manifest our intention of living our lives in a holistic way: a complete self.

6

The Power of
Movement

As mentioned previously, the movements of an individual with autistic spectrum disorder (ASD) or Asperger's Syndrome (AS) exhibit a disconnection of the mind from body. Their movements are uncoordinated, helter-skelter in appearance, and ineffective energetically and mechanically. In this chapter I will offer simple Pathfinder movement exercises in which the AS student can reclaim, through repetition and disciplined training, confidence in movement that is elegant, powerful, and effective.

Movement is the physical expression of the dynamic fusion of vision, intention, and planning. When I am working with any client, whether he be a 22-year-old AS individual developing a comprehension of the mechanics of basic running, or a 45-year-old woman starting up physical rehabilitation from a hip-joint surgery, my mentoring strategy for both is developed by going through the following three steps.

The first stage in the process is creating a vision—a visual expression—of the situation at hand. For example, the woman with hip rehabilitation will clearly be able to understand and "see" in her mind's eye the hip-joint region by using an anatomy book to illustrate where her hip joint is placed in relationship to her whole body, how the hip joint functions, and what its range of possible movement and restrictions are. Then she can visualize and understand what muscles need to be strengthened in order to support the hip area for effective alignment and recovery from the surgery. Being able to literally see the anatomy involved helps her to be more effective in rehabilitation.

Second, the intention behind the training or rehabilitation work is acknowledged between the two of us—in this case, the trainer and the client. Together we discuss and agree upon why we are doing it this way, why it is important to be disciplined in the training ideas being utilized, and more importantly, honoring the long-range plan of personal health.

The last component in developing movement in the body is planning— the development of a sound strategy that is feasible, acceptable, and realistic for a successful and empowering outcome. In my years as a dance teacher, a martial arts instructor, fitness trainer, and Pathfinder mentor, it is in this stage that I must draw from the virtues of vigilance and disciplined awareness and be carefully observant of my student or client's *true* evolution to the next level in the training process. In order for a mentor, teacher, or parent to command the situation when guiding or teaching the AS individual, it is crucial to identify what is truthfully obtainable in the moment. Poor planning damages the student's self-confidence, producing physical chaos and frustration. Instead, the mentor must support the AS individual in order to break the cycles of learned detrimental behaviors from their past disasters and move to a enlightened place of empowerment and pride while in the process of learning something new or challenging. This is especially important in motor planning, which is often a weakness for people with ASD. Without clear guidance, we are setting them up for failure.

The combined components of vision, intention, and planning become a singular fluid state of energetic and kinetic flow (from both learned and unlearned responses and behaviors) that the body executes in a flash upon receiving the command from the brain, resulting in the desired movement. After training and practice, it is a joy to observe my mentees when these components finally come together in smooth, coordinated, flowing movement.

A movement exercise is the stage where we put all the earlier training of breath, mind, and body together and test it out. I have observed that when my AS clients, especially the older males aged 18–25 years, achieve any level of proficiency in the Pathfinder movements, they begin to glow with an inner sense of satisfaction and pride that those around them, their parents and friends, pick up on immediately. The parents are quite familiar with the lack of energy and health awareness that their sons have displayed about their bodies and their outlook on life for years. Now they see their sons are actually walking upright with a new awareness of self and *relationship* to those around them. They recognize and respect their sons' abilities to persevere and to stay disciplined through the challenging stages of learning. Their sons have learned something about themselves that was once as alien to them as a foreign language: a new understanding of self through enhanced body awareness and confidence while in movement.

I have observed that, as an AS client finds success in movement, their new-found empowerment extends into a renewed positive outlook towards their whole life. For now that they are actually *moving*, they are also breaking out of their old cocoon of self-doubt, self-criticism, and self-loathing. They now have their body grounded and charged to really challenge some of the critical issues facing them—the same issues they had been avoiding for most of their life. Some of the critical issues demanding attention of the AS teen or young adult include achieving academic resolution, high-school graduation, obtaining a General Education Diploma and going to college, as well as post high-school transitional planning, applying and holding on to a job, moving away from home, driving a car, doing one's own laundry and shopping, living healthfully, and developing friends and relationships.

The Pathfinder teaching affirmation—"Movement disrupts stagnation"—is a mantra said over and over again by me to remind my clients and students that to move is to heal. To break old cycles, one has to move in order to generate the energy to break up inertia—the numbness of life and vitality. Many professionals as well as parents have noted that inertia is rampant among the ASD crowd, the "couch potato" or "computer gamer" "stay-at-home" phenomenon. Getting people to move affects all areas of their lives. "Movement disrupts stagnation."

The movements I offer are based on dance movement studies, movement improvisations, and martial arts. In martial arts, one trains so that the whole being moves from point "A" to point "B" as one complete piece with precision, grace, and power. The economy of movement is a concept taught in close combat techniques. To describe this in warriorship terms, the whole body involved in movement is critical to avoid personal injury and serious harm when faced with aggressive offensive movement from an attacker. In teaching weapons training to clients with the wooden sword, for instance, I point out that leaving part of yourself behind when moving—your leg or an arm—or leading with a part of your body—like your head, for instance—is an invitation for decapitation, having something severed from the body, or being inflicted with a serious wound. To be safe, you move as one.

"Moving as one piece"—one body—reinforces the concept of complete mind/body living: at all times being aware of the self in relation to what's happening in the environment.

The most simple example of "moving as one piece" is the mechanics of walking.

As a full-scholarship dance student at the Alvin Ailey School of American Dance in New York, during my break between dance classes I would sit on the stairs of the New York City public library on 5th Avenue and 42nd Street and watch people walk by. All types of people and all types of walking behaviors are to be observed on the streets of New York City at any given time. I watched, observed, and took notes on how people carried their bodies while walking. Being a student of dance and still learning how to hold my own body, watching others taught me much about myself.

Here are the basic behaviors in walking I have observed through the years. There are as many variations to the movement walking as there are snowflakes and individual grains of sand!

1. Walking with the head and torso positioned in front of the pelvis. This is where the person appears as if they are falling forwards while walking. In walking, the person is actually being propelled forward by this distribution of body weight forward of the center of balance: the pelvis towards the ball of the feet and toes. In a sense, this type of walker is literally, "ahead of themselves." Their thoughts are moving faster than their body can actually carry them. Hyper in energy and lacking in mindfulness, being "ahead of themselves," they walk into ambush (Figure 6.1).

2. Walking with the head and torso positioned behind or following the pelvis. With the weight of the head and torso behind the center of balance in the pelvis, this type of walker is heel heavy in stride and their contact to earth is jarring and stressful on the body. This type of walker is literally behind themselves, thinking of the past and what has happened while paying very little attention to the present moment. Here too the person falls prey, in this case for "falling behind." Isolated, they are easily ambushed (Figure 6.2).

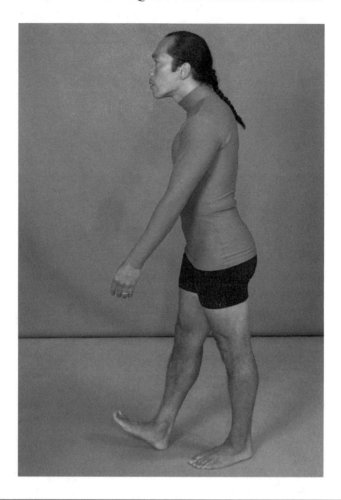

Figure 6.1 Walking with head in front of the body alignment

3. Leaning to one side walking. From injury, wearing purses and backpacks on one shoulder, work-related stress, or physical behavior learned at an early age and not corrected, the leaning to one side walker favors one leg or settles into one hip. Leaning to one side through the pelvis sends the head and torso in the opposite direction to maintain balance in the body. This type of walker often leans upon that same side hip and leg while in a stationary standing position.

4. Social behavioral walking and mimicking. As a child growing up in San Francisco during the early 1960s in a lower-class neighborhood, most of my friends were streetwise and would walk

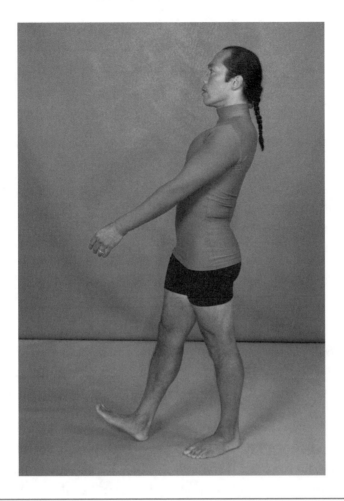

Figure 6.2 Walking with head behind the body alignment

with a strut-like-shuffle down the street. I would drag one foot slightly as I "did my thang" down the street with my buddies. I walked no differently than my Afro-American, Chicano, and Asian American buddies. It was a strut that came from listening to Motown recording artists and other "black music" of the time, which generated the feelings of being cool, invincible, extremely cocky and bold. The music shaped our physical expressions and language. My walk defined who I was in my society: a young inner-city boy, mildly defiant and rebellious against authority. Only the styles have changed as American society experienced the disco era of the 1980s, the rap "gangsta" scene of the 1990s and now the hip-hop age of the new millennium. The big difference is that with the advent of better technology for television and computers since the 1980s, social physical behaviors and fads found in music have become more accessible and obtainable by the general masses. Now we have the "melting pot of styles" generation—where white, black, red, and yellow young people are shuffling and hanging out of their bodies all over the world. It is extremely funny and amazing to see a youth in Thailand strut the American "ghetto thang." However, my concern is that those stylized manners of walking can lead to poor alignment and stress on the body if they become long-term habits. These mannerisms may create a negative impression in some situations such as a job interview.

5. ASD walking. In my observations of the movement of walking with my ASD clients throughout the years, I have noted some of the following types:

    o   Balls of the feet walking—this type of walking has bouncy up-down stride. In running, the movement is an inhibiting up-down stride rather moving forward and gaining speed (Figure 6.3).

    o   Outside rim of foot walking—walking more on the outside rim of the foot, the walker stresses the ankles and creates a wobbly stride. Indications of outside wearing of the shoe will be present.

    o   Heavy heel walking—clumpy, heavy, and loud is the heavy heel walker. Lagging behind and having a hard time catching up is this type of walker.

Proper walking exercise

Let us now study proper walking mechanics. Proper walking means that the walker is pro-active in the process—aware in the mind and engaged with the body to produce a walking that is confident and healthy. The following exercise is one I enjoy teaching. It is a real eye-opener for my clients as I mirror and demonstrate their various walking movements. These clients have no clue as to how they appear until they watch my imitations. After these humbling, yet playful demonstrations of their old walking habits, they are ready to learn how to improve.

Instructor's notes:

- This exercise is best done in a cleared area in which the students can walk across the room. Use the diagonal length of the room because it affords the longest distance to experiment on.

- If leading this exercise, the following is to be read out loud:

    1. Everyone, please stand and take three breaths of *misogi* to clear the slate in your minds, and to settle down. You may learn something new from a calm place.

    2. Please line up here in double file. Thank you.

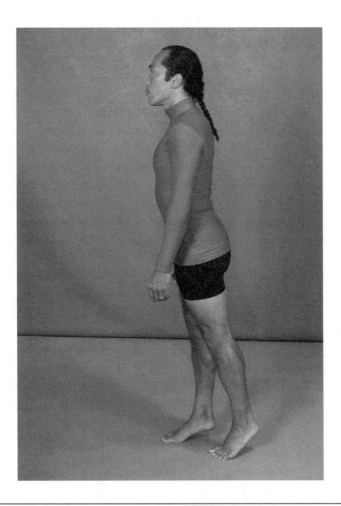

Figure 6.3 "Ball of the feet" walking

3. Now we are going to practice walking in a way that will demonstrate the concepts we have learned earlier about posture, presence, and extension of our minds and bodies.

4. Let's quickly review the points of alignment:

    o   Live feet: tripod points in the feet activated. Visualization: Imagine your feet are three-pronged plugs and earth is the outlet. Push into these points downwards, as if you are "plugging" into earth.

    o   Soft relaxed ankles.

    o   Knees soft and flexible—they are the "shock absorbers" of the body.

    o   The pelvic girdle "floats" right on top of two legs. This speaks about releasing old tension in the buttocks and lower back.

    o   Belly breathing into the lower abdominal area. Allow the lungs to inflate and deflate naturally. Keep your facial mask relaxed, especially the muscles around the mouth and eyes.

    o   The sunburst points. Visualization: Visualize a sunburst—energy expanding outwardly from a central point. There are two points to consider—one sunburst point is located on the breast bone or sternum area and the other sunburst point is located between the shoulder blades.

    o   Relax the neck and shoulder muscles—because you are now aware of dropping your breath energy into the belly.

    o   Finally, bring the head back to neutral. Neutral is a place where your head sits comfortably right on top of the neck.

5. Is everyone ok on the points of alignment? Good.

6. Now we are going to move your aligned posture in your body while walking.

7. First, to illustrate what walking with posture feels like, let's do a movement game where we show all the different ways people walk out of alignment.

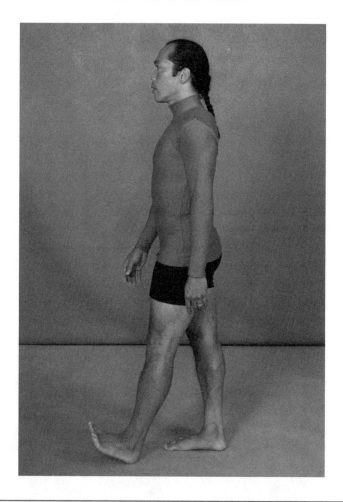

Figure 6.4 Step through and repeat: heel—ball—toes

8. Ok. So let us try walking with our upper body's balance on the front of our feet. Got it? Good. Notice how this affects your standing posture (demonstrate) (Figure 6.1).

9. Now, two at a time, please walk across the room while keeping the balance of your body towards the front of your feet. (Give the first pair ten paces before the next pair begins.) Notice anything you feel or experience while walking across the room. Having fun is ok while experimenting with walking, yet going "out there" is not—that's annoying. (Note: teachers please take visual note on how they are walking: What is their head-to-pelvis relationship? What is happening to their shoulders? How

effective is their walking stride in balance and in fluidity? Have them return to the original beginning point.)

10. (Everyone is done crossing twice) Great! Anyone pick up anything—any funny feelings or sensations in your bodies or thoughts—while walking with your weight more in the front of your center of balance? Anyone want to share what you experienced?

11. Ok. Now, let us try walking across the room where the upper body's balance point is more on our heels, our heads are now behind our center of balance, yet we are still moving forward in our walking stride. (Demonstrate for them and have them cross

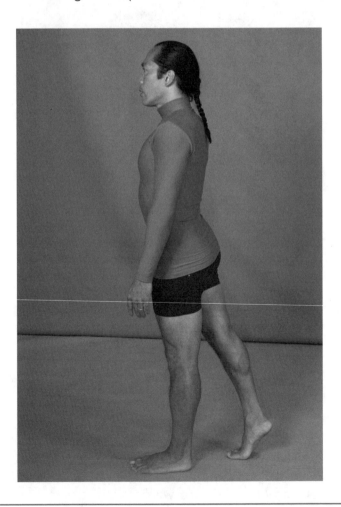

Figure 6.5 Push through the back foot: toe—ball—heel—shift weight to front foot to move forward

the floor twice to experiment and study, as well as having fun in a focussed, relaxed way (Figure 6.2).)

12. Nice! Anyone pick up anything—any funny feelings or sensations in your bodies or thoughts—while walking with your weight more in the back of your center of balance? Anyone want to share what you experienced?

13. Well, if we can walk with our body's weight in the front and in the back of our center of balance, we should be able to move our balance to each side—left and right.

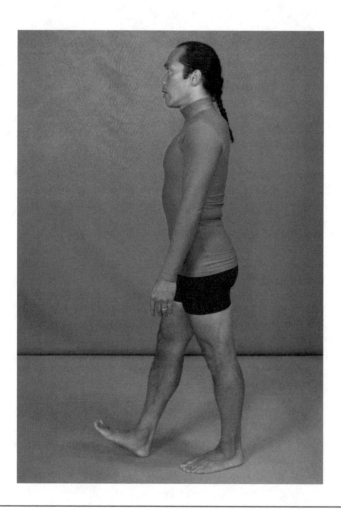

Figure 6.6 After stepping forward—go through the foot as you contact the ground:
heel—ball—toes

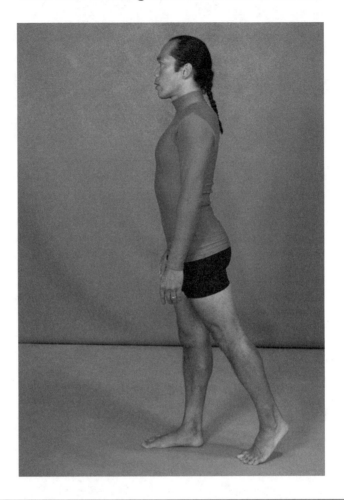

Figure 6.7 Shift weight to the front foot and now push through the back foot: toes—ball—heel

14. With that in mind, let's place our upper body posture from the waist up slightly past the balance point on our right side. (Demonstrate for them and have them cross the floor twice, in a focussed, relaxed way.)

15. Let's now place our upper body posture from the waist up slightly past the balance point on our left side. (Demonstrate for them and have them cross the floor twice, in a focussed relaxed way).

16. All right. Now let's discover walking in alignment.

17. First, please arrange your body using the points of alignment.

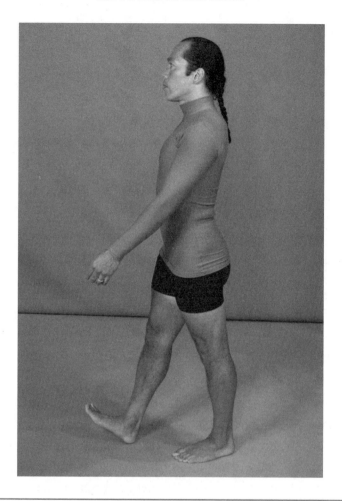

Figure 6.8 Walking in a "grounded" way

18. Now, with your body in alignment, the movement of walking stays connected to earth through your feet and you maintain posture while moving (Figures 6.4, 6.5, 6.6, 6.7).

19. Remember, as we try this out, to use our breathing awareness so we can keep extending energy through our feet—connecting us to earth.

20. As we walk in this "grounded way," be alert to extending energy through our sunburst points in our upper bodies. We are not walking with our shoulders slumped and rolled forward (Figure 6.8).

21. Let's try it out. Two at a time—walking with energy and extension.

22. Now that everyone has done it, I observed some of you walking on the balls of your feet like this (demonstrate).

23. Let's all walk through our feet in a very effective way. When walking forward we would like to use the mechanics of motion by which we walk heel—ball—toes through both feet. This will allow us to use our ankles differently and correctly to help prevent injuring our ankles while we are at play or activity.

24. Ok. Let us all try walking now through our feet: heel—ball—toes.

25. Great! Everyone looked great. Walking with energy allows us to protect our back and correct our alignment.

26. Please do three breaths of *misogi* to finish. Thank you everyone for doing the exercise.

Three basic *aikido* movements

There are three basic movements in the Japanese martial art *aikido*. The three basic *aikido* movements are *irimi, tenkan,* and *kaiten*. These three movements can be combined in numerous variations.

Aikido is based on the sword. In ancient times, attention and intention in the combat strategy using the Japanese sword was very simple: one cut—one kill. Owning the "line of fire" was the course of strategy: no running away and saving oneself. There was no time to engage one enemy when surrounded by many. One stood and dominated one's enemy with the intention of "one cut—one kill." A Japanese warrior or *samurai* faced life and death with fearlessness. The line of fire is a vector—the direction in which energy is coming at you. This energy in martial training can be in the form of a punch, push, kick, head butt, or any focussed energy coming at you that you would like to avoid. One of the first key concepts of *aikido* strategy that beginners need to understand is that the opening movement in a connection with an attacker creates options in tight situations by first moving oneself off the line of fire; second blending with the oncoming energy of the attack; and, last finding harmonious resolution by using, or returning oncoming energy back upon the attacker.

The following photos (Figures 6.9, 6.10, 6.11) illustrate moving off the line of fire using wooden swords. I will show the exercise with student Nate.

To my mentees, I use the martial attack as a metaphor for any conflict that may be challenging in their normal daily lives. For instance, I might say to my mentees:

> The conflict you are challenged with could be a fellow student who is annoying you in school, or a very difficult writing assignment that is due soon yet you have not started it because you are anxious about it and procrastinated, or maybe you are having to deal with a unexpected transition or change in your routine, or dealing with unexpected stress load, or dealing with your current time management quandaries, learning to drive,

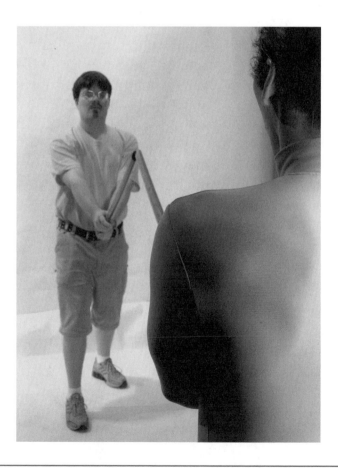

Figure 6.9 Nate (facing) is on the line of fire facing me. We both have wooden swords or bokkens

going for a job interview for the first time, or learning something new and the process of learning brings out your old fears. You will learn that challenges are best approached by flowing and blending with them, rather than bumping, bashing and creating conflict. Blending and flowing with challenge makes life easier for you!

These three movements, most especially the movement of *irimi*, awaken the whole mind/body of my mentees with awareness and purpose in action.

I teach the importance of moving "off the line of fire" with an *aiki-shinai*, a sword of bamboo wrapped in leather. The *shinai* allows for reality training without injury should the mentee not move off line of fire in a exercise—a very valuable lesson in illustrating conflict resolution.

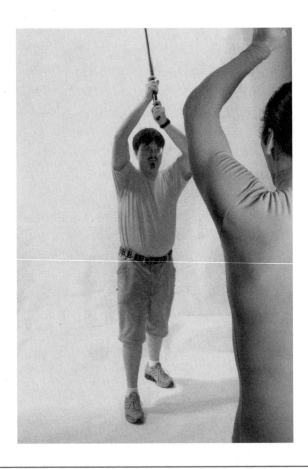

Figure 6.10 Our swords are raised and I will strike at Nate on the line of fire and not tracking him

Using the *shinai* also shows if the student is completely off the line of fire by touching or lightly striking a shoulder, a hand, or maybe a dragging leg or foot left on the "line." The lesson is that the *whole mind and body* must get off the line of fire in order to be safe and ready to respond to whatever happens next.

In the *irimi* movement, a person either enters strongly off the line of fire or enters on the line of fire and dominates the oncoming energy.

In the second movement *tenkan*, one enters off the line of fire and turns the whole body.

And in the third movement, *kaiten*, one enters off the line of fire and pivots the whole body.

In all the movements, the person has a choice to get off the line of fire and avoid conflict or, in the case of *irimi*, the person may also choose to

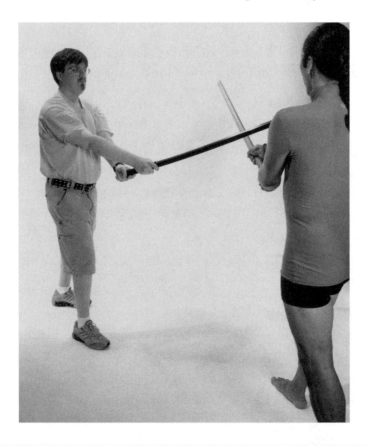

Figure 6.11 Nate blends with my sword attack without fear by moving off the line of fire. He maintains connection to me with focus, awareness, and intention

decisively own the line of fire and defuse the energy coming at them with faith and fearlessness. The key word here is *choice*—a person has the choice to mindfully decide to do something that preserves their life with harmony and without conflict. The choice is to do something differently—to break old patterns.

The three basic movements of *aikido*

Instructor's notes:

- This exercise is best done in a cleared area in which the students can move safely and without hindrance.

- If leading this exercise, the following is to be read out loud:

Irimi (e-re-me)—"*to enter*"

1. Please begin by doing three breaths of misogi to clear the slate and get ready to learn something new. Good! Let's begin.

2. The first idea to think about is when you are moving and learning, please stay relaxed even if you are finding the exercise challenging. We will do the movements slowly and learn without stress and anxiety.

3. All martial movement is done without a sense of fear or doubt. Once you understand the movements, allow yourself to become confident and fearless.

4. Ready? Ok, let us all start with the left foot forward so we are on the same page.

5. Arms down relaxed by your sides.

6. It is important to understand the difference between sliding and stepping. In stepping, the back foot comes forward and alternates with the front as in walking. In sliding, you move forward in the direction of the foot in front of you, keeping the same foot in front when finished moving. (Try sliding and stepping movements numerous times on both sides—left and right foot forward—until everyone is comfortable and confident with the movements.)

7. Watch me first demonstrate the first *aikido* movement *irimi* (Figure 6.12). Do not do—please watch. (Demonstrate and explain the line of fire and the importance of getting off the line to avoid conflict.)

8. Ok, try this with me slowly at first. First, inhale now—and, as you exhale, slide forward off the line of fire in the direction of your front foot, not changing feet, the same foot will remain forward, and bring your arms up to chest level, in front of your sunburst point, and extend out your fingertips (Figure 6.13).

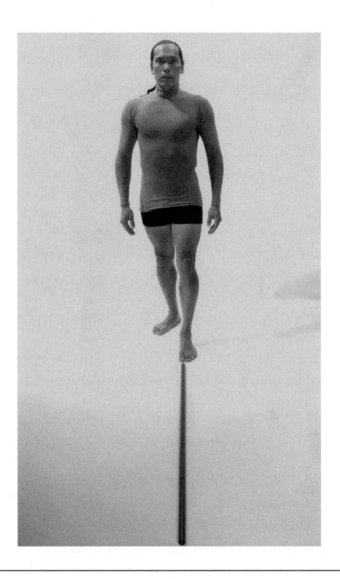

Figure 6.12 Irimi with left foot forward using a staff to show the line of fire

9. Slide back to your starting position on the inhale—arms come back to your sides—and on the exhale slide forward again, raising your arms and extending out your fingertips.

10. The important idea here is to move as one piece—avoid leading with your head or your pelvis. Bring your whole body off the line of fire and safely avoid any incoming energy. We want to move as one piece and not leave any part of our bodies behind on the line of fire.

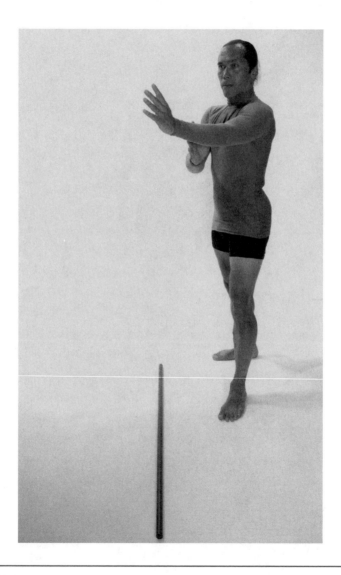

Figure 6.13 Slide forward in the direction of the front foot. Finish with arms extending energy through them

11. Another note is, when you are finished with the *irimi* movement, remember to be fully charged and extending through your body. This is a very important time to practice extending and using your body with energy and purpose.

12. Let's now do our other side. Good, right foot forward now (Figures 6.14, 6.15).

13. Do this numerous times.

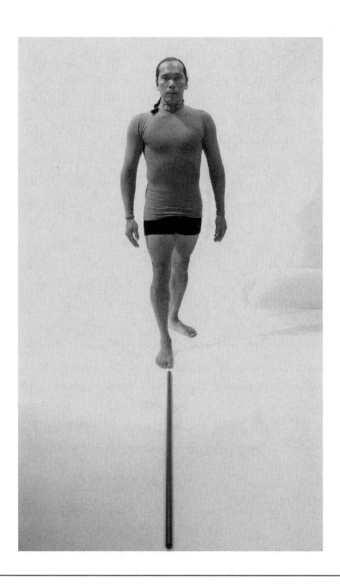

Figure 6.14 Irimi with right foot forward

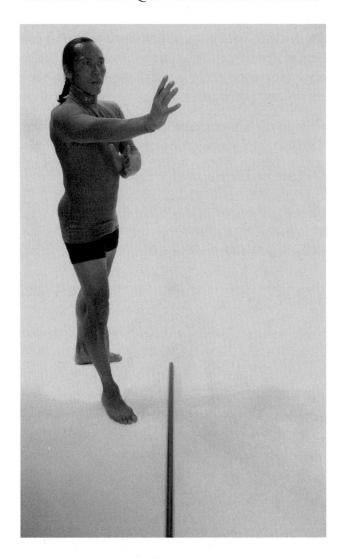

Figure 6.15 Sliding forward towards the right side—finishing with arms extending energy through them

Tenkan (ten-con)—*"to turn"*:

1. Please take three breaths of *misogi* to clear out and settle down for the next movement.

2. Ok, let's try the next movement called *tenkan*. Like the first movement, *irimi*, we want to blend with energy coming at us with confidence and without fear.

3. The *tenkan* movement is done by sliding off the line of fire first in the direction of your front foot, then pivoting on the front foot and drawing a three-quarter circle on the ground with your back foot. We want to move as one piece and not leave any part of our bodies behind on the line of fire.

4. Let us all start with the left foot forward.

5. Inhale. Raise your left arm and hand as if you are going to shake someone's hand but with your palm facing down. Curl your fingers of your left hand towards your belly and (Figure 6.16)…

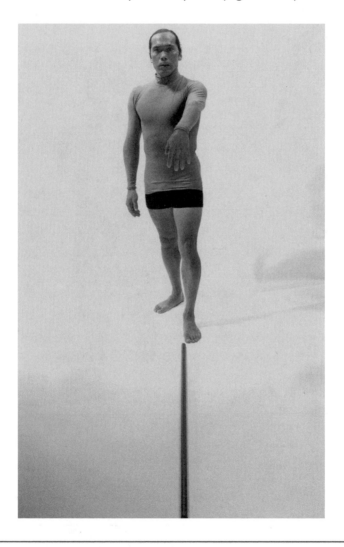

Figure 6.16 Tenkan with left foot forward. Begin by pointing your left hand towards your belly

6. ...as you exhale, slide forward off the line of fire with your left foot. With your back foot—your right foot—draw a three-quarter circle on the ground behind you like your back foot is a compass. You will finish with the right foot still behind you (Figures 6.17. 6.18, 6.19).

7. When finished, both of your palms are facing up and extending energy through your fingers like beams of light shooting out of each of your fingertips (Figure 6.20).

8. Again, like the *irimi* movement, move as one piece leaving nothing on the line. In all movements again, please keep your posture and move with your breath.

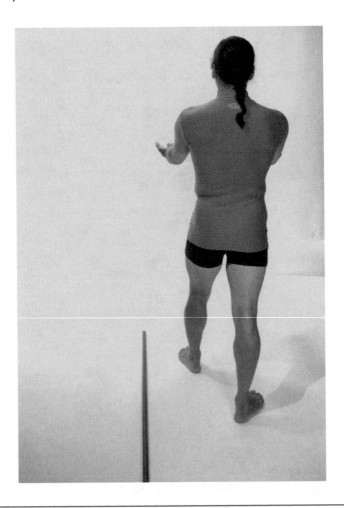

Figure 6.17 Slide forward to left of the line of fire and your back foot will draw a half circle on the ground and finish behind you

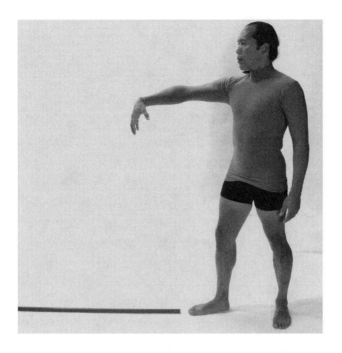

Figure 6.18 Side view of tenkan

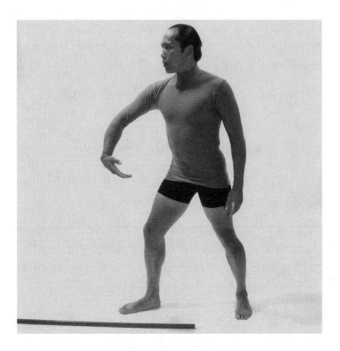

Figure 6.19 Side view of tenkan, slide in...

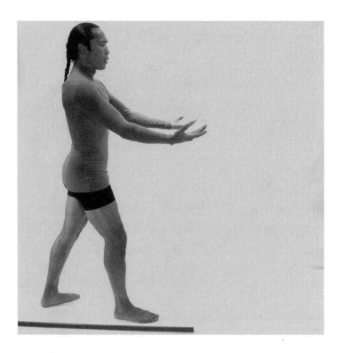

Figure 6.20 Finish position of tenkan with extension of energy

9. Do this side numerous times noting that everyone is getting it and is relaxed about doing the movement. Do not change to the other side until everyone is doing the movement. Remember: slow down, teach and learn without stress!

10. Good! Now let us switch feet and do the other side.

Kaiten (kai-ten)—*"to pivot"*

1. Please do three breaths of *misogi*, to clear your minds and bodies for the last *aikido* movement called *kaiten*.

2. Remember, everyone: we are studying movement to open the energy in our bodies and also to learn to get off the line of fire or deal with any conflict safely. In a moment we will discuss how these *aikido* exercises can help you in your daily lives.

3. Ok, here we go! *Kaiten*, is the last basic *aikido* movement. Like the first two movements, *irimi* and *tenkan*, we want to safely avoid conflict directed at us without creating conflict in return. We want to move as

one piece, not leaving anything behind—any part of our bodies on the line of fire.

4. Let us begin with our left foot forward again (Figure 6.21).

5. As in *irimi* and *tenkan* movements, we want to slide forward off the line of fire in the direction of our front foot—in this case our left foot—on our inhale (Figure 6.22).

6. And as we exhale—leaving our feet where they are—open or pivot our hips to face the direction we just came from, allowing our feet to pivot, facing the same direction as our hips (Figure 6.23).

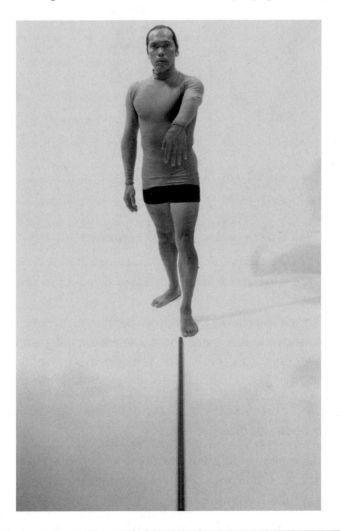

Figure 6.21 Opening position is the same as tenkan, in this case left foot forward left hand lifted

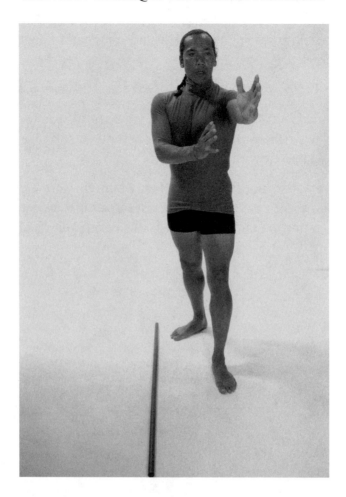

Figure 6.22 Slide forward off the line of fire in the direction of your front foot

7. To finish, extend energy through our hands and our whole bodies. We want to move as one piece and not leave anything—any part of our bodies—behind on the line of fire (do the movement numerous times).

8. *Kaiten* movement is very quick like *irimi*. We enter strongly and then quickly open our hips and pivot.

9. This movement is different from *tenkan*, because we will finish with the back foot in front when we are done moving. Remember, in *tenkan* we finish with the same foot front as we started.

10. Ok, let us try it on the other side now. Here we go! (Do the movement numerous times.)

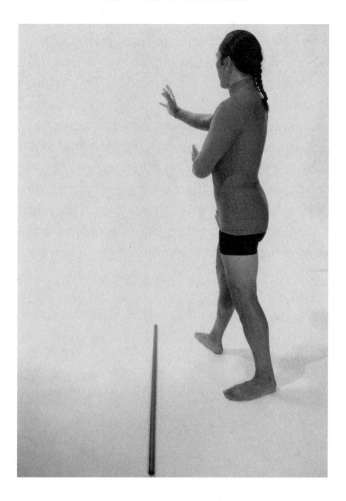

Figure 6.23 Open or pivot your hips to face the direction you just came from, allowing your feet to pivot, facing the same direction as your hips

11. Excellent! Now let us review the movements. (Please do all three movements now, cleaning up the movements and making sure everyone is safe and learning without stress.)

12. Everyone, great job everyone staying cool and relaxed while we learned these movements.

13. Please do three breaths of *misogi* to finish. Thank you.

Instructor's notes: Now lead a discussion on how the *aikido* movements can teach us about avoiding conflict in our daily lives and dealing with our challenges by blending and staying grounded. Through movements you can teach the concepts of conflict resolution. Give examples of how to blend and harmonize with conflict by using our language, our thoughts and actions. Examples of the wrong way, not blending, and the right way, blending, can be helpful in illustrating this. Students may enjoy acting out the right way of blending and the wrong way (running away, escalating, being overly defensive) in a variety of situations that they themselves come up with. Ask them to volunteer examples of problems they are facing in their lives, and have them act out blending compared to clashing head on.

7

The Rites of Passage

Honoring the Rites of Passage

The 20th century has brought into human consciousness the ability to see and create way beyond what was humanly capable in our past. As our world leaped and bounded through technical and medical achievements, we of this modern advanced society are now seeing some negative effects of such speed at which our society is rushing ahead upon our young men and women. Today the 21st century quickness of our lives is displayed in our instantaneous global communication anywhere in the world through our wireless phones and small mobile personal computers. Boy, we are moving real fast!

Picking up the newspaper, we observed a constant reporting of the frightening display of violence, debauchery, and suicide committed by adolescents that was prevalent throughout the 1990s and continuous into our present 21st-century society. An epidemic of poor eating habits and inactive behavior fueled by a need to sit and be stimulated by a screen has taken over much of the attention of today's youths.

As someone who has worked with adolescents since the 1980s I have observed and experienced how adolescents would struggle to keep up with their ever-changing environment of what is in and what is out, as far as fads and styles are concerned.

It is not like these issues did not occur in my adolescent years of the late 1960s and early 1970s, or any generation before mine. It is just that today's stimulations and arousal factors are a heck of a lot faster, glitterier, flashier, more excessive and expensive, and more easily accessible. The culture is global and there are not many things that can't be researched, found out, sold and bought, downloaded and enjoyed by the privacy of a personal computer in a four-walled room behind a door.

For adolescents with autistic spectrum disorder (ASD) or Asperger's Syndrome (AS) today's distractions can take a devastating tone in social, academic, and health development.

There is a void, the emptiness, in our adolescents' consciousness of personal growth, maturity, and connection to our greater society. For some adolescents their connection with other age groups in their communities has widened to a place of being strangers. Like ships passing in the night, the different age groups miss out on each other's strengths and assets that could be shared. A noted country like Japan, who as a nation treasured a custom of responsibility and respect to the Elder, has seen a major decline in such behavior displayed by their adolescent Japanese to their elder Japanese counterparts.

In ages past, most cultures had the Coming of Age or the Rites of Passage as a built-in program in the society that maintained and created a bridge of connection from a boy to a man and a girl to a woman. This transition marked a new adult role and sense of responsibility to and for their community. This special ritual of Rites of Passage occurred during the age of 12–13 years old generally. In some cultures 16 years old marks this special time of transition.

Today, in indigenous cultures unaffected by modern age technology, the Rite of Passage is still important. In some cultures, the young boy is "kidnapped" from the mother's home by the male elders and warriors of the tribe to be initiated to the adult male psyche and world. This male world perspective, with its manners, behaviors, and conduct, showed the newly initiated boy-man what was expected from him now. The transition to adulthood culminates in a new position within the tribe. For example, the initiated young man may be given a spear and entrusted to guard the tribe's livestock. I mean, "There ain't no messin' around here!"

In this situation, the young man is now part of the tribe's functioning strength, and a possible direct participant to the tribe's future through marriage and procreation.

The stakes are higher for the newly initiated young warrior and rightly so. He is not a young boy living behind "The Mother" anymore. He is now a man among men behaving and conducting himself as a peer among peers.

The mentee is now *mentored* in the skills of the men of their society and taught the virtues of being an adult male. He is held responsible for his actions and words. He is valued for his deeds as well as his intentions. His actions reflect upon a tribe's values and rituals. He represents his tribe, his society, and his community. Now can you picture anything like this occurring in the US of A? Get out of here!

The metamorphosis that occurs through traditional Rites of Passage ritual can at times be a very shocking rude awakening—a real eye-opening experience to free one from the comfort zone of one's past life. Some rituals involve the whole tribe/family while others are a solitary experience guided by an elder or mentor.

I found in my own work with adolescents that the inclusion of the Rites of Passage as a concept or story evoked a sense of clarified purpose and intention of action for making personal changes for the mentee in training.

For example, I use the Rites of Passage idea to explain the social behavioral changes that need to occur for the young man who is still acting like a young boy.

Noting for the ASD teen that a young man initiated in an indigenous tribe in a land like Africa or Asia would be given a lot of responsibility in their tribe or community, such as guarding the herd from lions or looking after the elderly of their tribe or community, is a very powerful example of personal growth from boy to man. Such responsibility required the maturity, courage, and wisdom of a young man not of a young boy. Using this simple and obvious example in an indigenous people's experience really opens some of my ASD and AS students' eyes.

I explained how the cushy life in Western modern society which we live in creates a void for the Rite of Passage to be experienced in their lives. I described how a Western young person is a bit soft skinned and babied and spoiled compared to their counterparts throughout the world. I use this comparison to appeal to their untapped desire to explore proper age-appropriate behavior and manners. I do not expect any of them to change overnight. The seed planted from this place by my work as a mentor and teacher can develop.

The student's maturity will of course evolve with age and more experience. The student with ASD will also mature and evolve regardless of their so-called disabilities.

I have helped adolescent males aged 11 and 12 of single-parent mothers develop their personal Rites of Passage ceremonies. These ceremonies crossed cultural, religious, and social boundaries. These young boys on their way to be young men created unique Rites of Passage ceremonies that fitted them personally, and therefore their ceremonies meant something real to them and were not just ritual gestures that had only fluff value.

Part of the process these young boys studied were the paths of maturity and what that called for in being pro-active in their personal growth and transformation. In a wonderful way, they understood what it meant to be a little bit older and a little bit wiser in an unpretentious way.

In the classroom, I use the teachings of the process of the Rites of Passage as a reminder of what I will expect from my students in terms of their age-appropriate behavior, self-discipline, and self-awareness. This is a challenge for your "neuro-typical" adolescent. For an ASD or AS student, it may be a big stretch for them to comprehend and want to achieve this challenge.

I have witnessed a core awakening in my students especially the older ones—the 15–22-year-olds. They do not stop playing computer or video games—that's not the point. Nor do they ditch their plastic action figures. The core-awakened ASD individual matures and develops the self-referred sense of responsibility of their decisions. This speaks about a quality of mindfulness to pause in one's actions and to take the time to investigate and weigh out the consequences of reasonable options—to make the right safe choice. The mentee now understands their place in life, which is to grow mature and express their potential whatever that may be to the highest degree of truth, compassion, honor, and vision.

In the lives of the young adolescents, creating opportunities to understand the virtues of the Rites of Passage, and thereby opening the door to the positive challenging according to its meanings, values, and teachings, will go a long way in reclaiming a way of being pro-active, empowered, and significant in their personal lives and ultimately their personal relationships within their community.

Bibliography

Almedia, B. (1986) *Capoeira—A Brazilian Art Form.* Berkeley, CA: North Atlantic Books.

Asperger, H. (1944) *Autism and Asperger's Syndrome.* Cambridge, England: Cambridge University Press.

Attwood, T. (2006) *The Complete Guide to Asperger's Syndrome.* London: Jessica Kingsley Publishers.

Eckstein, G. (1970) *The Body Has a Head.* New York: Harper and Row.

Moore, R. and Gillette, D. (1990) *King, Warrior, Magician, Lover.* New York: HarperCollins Publishers.

Perkins, J., Ridenhour, A. and Kovsky, M. (2000) *Attack Proof—The Ultimate Guide to Personal Protection.* Champaign, IL: Human Kinetics.

Pressfield, S. (1998) *The Gates of Fire: An Epic Novel of the Battle of Thermopylae.* New York: Bantam.

Rachlin, H. (2000) *The Science of Self-Control.* Cambridge, MA: Harvard University Press.

Saito, M. (1973) *Traditional Aikido,* Vols 1–4. Tokyo: Sugawara Martial Arts Institute/Japan Publications.

Saotome, M. (1993) *The Principles of Aikido.* Boston: Shambhala Publications, Inc.

Shioda, G. (1968) *Dynamic Aikido.* Tokyo: Kodansha International.

Stevens, J. (1999) *The Essence of Aikido: Spiritual Teachings of Morihei Ueshiba.* Tokyo: Kodansha International.

Stevens, J. with Krenner, W. (1999) *Training with the Master: Lessons with Morihei Ueshiba.* Boston: Shambhala Publications, Inc.

Stevens, J. and Rinjiro, S. (1984) *Aikido: The Way of Harmony.* Boston: Shambhala Publications, Inc.

Talbot, M. (1992) *The Holographic Universe.* New York: HarperPerennial.

Ueshiba, K. (1997) *The Spirit Of Aikido.* Tokyo: Kodansha International.

Ueshiba, M. (1991) *Budo—Teachings of the Founder of Aikido.* Tokyo: Kodansha International.

Ueshiba, M. (1992) *The Art of Peace* (translated by John Stevens). Boston: Shambhala Publications, Inc.

Ueshiba, M. (1997) *Budo Training in Aikido.* Tokyo: Sugawara Martial Arts Institute/Japan Publications.

Yamada, Y. (1981) *The New Aikido Complete.* West Hanover, MA: Halliday Lithographs.

Index

Page number in *italics* refer
to figures

adolescents 24, 64–5,
    88–9, 94, 104
  breathing 47–8, 59–60
  Rites of Passage 37,
    143–6
aiki-shinai sword 128–9
aikido 34–5, 36, 102
  three basic movements
    126–42
alignment
  basic points 68–72, 79,
    120
  walking 115–26, *116,*
    117, 119, 121, 122,
    123, 124, 125
  see also posture
Asperger, H. 16, 64
Attwood, T. 57, 60

backpacks and posture 65,
    66, 67
balancing

art of 104–6
  basic exercise 106–9,
    107, 108, 109
  checklist 110–11
Baum, W. 19–20
behavior
  analysis 19–20, 24
  changing 48–9
  social behavioral
    walking and
    mimicking 116–18
belly breathing 44–6
  alignment 72, *73,* 79,
    120
  posture exercise 89–92,
    90, 91, 93
berserker warrior 27–8
body awareness 65–8,
    110, 113–14
"BodyKi" 22, 24, 25
breath awareness 39–40,
    59–60, 67
breathing exercises 40–4
  see also belly breathing;
    misogi breathing

calmness *see* mindfulness
character mimic exercise
    100
"chattering mind" 48,
    55–7
childhood abuse 22, 65,
    88
"clear vase" visualization
    24, 60–3
"clearing the mind space"
    visualization 58–60
"clearing the slate:
    emptying the cup"
    47–9
comfort zones, pushing
    beyond 31, 32–3, 38,
    101, 145
communication 84–5
conflict, martial attack as
    metaphor 127–8, 142

dancing
  balance 105–6, 110
  extension 101
  healing injuries 22

mindfulness 59, 60
movement 34–5, 44,
    114, 115
posture 92–4

Eastern and Western
    philosophies 18–19,
    22
Eckstein, G. 18
energy flow 72, 88, 92
entering see irimi
exercises
    aikido 130–42
    balancing 106–9, 107,
        108, 109
    basic floor (for upper
        back) 89–92, 90, 91,
        93
    basic movements
        130–42, 131, 132,
        133 ,134, 135, 136,
        137, 138, 139, 140,
        141
    belly breathing 45–6,
        45, 46
    character mimic 100
    "making gold coins"
        81–4, 110, 82, 83
    "sitting on your throne"
        94–8, 95, 96, 97, 98
    "standing your ground"
        78–80, 80
    "unbreakable arm" 102,
        103, 104
    walking 118–26, 116,
        117, 119, 121, 122,
        123, 124, 125

extension 101–4
eye gaze 79, 106, 110
"eye of the hurricane"
    exercise 33–6, 34

floor exercise (for upper
    back) 89–92, 90, 91,
    93

Gillette, D. 27
gravity
    collapsed posture 88
    honoring 81–4
    groundedness 84–6

head and neck alignment
    72, 76, 77, 78
healer warrior 27, 28–9
heroes 29, 31, 100
holistic approach 16, 21–5

intention in movement
    training 112–13
irimi 126, 128, 129–30
    exercise 130–4, 131,
        132, 133, 134
kaiten 126, 129
    exercise 13–41, 139,
        140, 141,
kohais–sempai relationship
    36–8
Krishnamurti, J. 19

"making gold coins"
    exercise 81–4, 110,
    82, 83

martial arts see aikido;
    warriorship
mentoring 11, 20
    core concepts 21–38
    relationship 9–10, 36–8,
        84–6
mimicking 100, 116–18
mind/body model 21–5
mindfulness 59–60
    and "chattering mind"
        48, 55–7
    "eye of the hurricane"
        exercise 33–6, 34
    see also misogi breathing;
        visualizations
misogi breathing 35–6,
    47–9
    alignment 78, 79, 80,
        81, 84, 126
    balancing 106, 110
    movement with 50–4
    posture 89, 94, 96
    presence 100, 102
Moore, R. 27
movement 112–15
    aikido 126–42
    with misogi breathing
        50–4
    walking 115–26

physical development
    17–18, 19, 64–5
pivoting see kaiten
planning in movement
    training 113
point of contact 9–10
posture 87–98

body awareness 65–8,
110, 113–14
see also alignment
presence 98–100
presence awareness 99
pro-active sitting 94–8
pro-active standing 72

Rachlin, H. 20
relationship 9–10, 36–8,
84–6
Rites of Passage 37,
143–6

sacredness 10, 21–2, 23
samurais 35, 47, 126
self–awareness 111,
113–14
sempai–kohai relationship
36–8
shinai sword 128–9
"sitting on your throne"
exercise 94–8, *95, 96,
97, 98*
social behavioral walking
and mimicking
116–18
spirituality 19, 22–3
"standing your ground"
exercise 78–80, *80*
sunburst points 72, *74, 75,
79,* 120

teenagers *see* adolescents
tenkan 126, 129
exercise 13–8, *135, 136,
137, 138*

therapeutic approaches
14–16
trauma
childhood abuse and 22,
65, 88
memory of 56, 61
trust 36–8
turning *see tenkan*

Ueshiba, M. 35
"unbreakable arm" exercise
102, *103, 104*

vision in movement
training 112, 113
visualizations
alignment exercises
68–9, 72, 78–9, 81,
120
"clear vase" 24, 60–3
"clearing the mind
space" 58–60
posture exercise 95
white light 49–54

walking 115–18
exercise 118–26
warrior stance *80*
warriorship 10–11, 15,
20, 21–2
archetype 25–33
and heroes 29, 31, 100
movement 114–15
Rites of Passage 144–5
samurais 35, 47, 126
Western and Eastern
philosophies 18–19,
22

white light visualization
49–54
withdrawn presence 99